THE SPANISH FLU

History Of The 1918 Great Influenza Born From
H1N1 Virus. The Deadliest Pandemic That The
Human Race Has Faced And Overcome

By
Bryan Anderson

CONTENTS

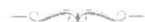

Introduction

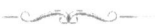

Influenza is a virus that belongs to the Ortho-myxoviridae family. It contains an enveloped virion, which includes a genome made from eight single-stranded negative-sense RNA segments that code for 10 or 11 referred proteins. For example, surface glycoproteins hemagglutinin (HA) and neuraminidase (NA), matrix and ion-channel proteins (M1 and M2), RNA polymerase subunits (PB1, PB2, and PA), nucleoprotein (NP), and nonstructural proteins (NS1 and NS2/NEP), using a few strains encoding another proapoptotic protein, PB1-F2. Reassortment among the flu virus genome segments is visible and it happens frequently. This phenomenon gives rise to mixtures of different subtypes of NA and HA that circulate in host populations. Waterfowl are believed to be the normal reservoirs of the influenza virus nonetheless; the virus is known to infect a lot of different hosts, such as humans, swine, horse, puppy, etc., along with a vast array of avian species. A comprehensive understanding of any pathogen, such as flu virus, necessitates comprehension of how variations in the arrangement of the pathogen genome (genotype) are expressed. This is required as it assists in understanding the differences from the operational qualities of the pathogen (phenotype). It's well-known that flu virus sequences constantly grow by accumulating mutations via a procedure called "genetic drift," where arrangement variants are introduced with the virus's low-fidelity polymerase. These are chosen to maintain significant structural and functional protein traits while trying to evade the host immune system. Comparative

1

genomics research has largely been limited to phylogenetic evaluation of whole-genome sections or statistical institutions of sequence variants at single residue ranks and their impacts on specific phenotypic attributes. Nonetheless, these methods of genomics have limitations. The analysis doesn't consider the effect of genomic residues on the phenotype of attention. Section analysis doesn't highlight the areas responsible for its effect. Additionally, although the ancestry of hereditary variations caused by the cumulative consequences of development can be shown from the phylogenetic tree topology, phenotypic changes arising from convergent evolution aren't shown through phylogenetic tree foliage. Sequence variations may additionally affect virus traits, which might not be subjected to powerful natural selective pressures from the reservoir host. For instance, it could measure the host range specificity of interspecies transmissibility modified with replication virulence and pathogenicity in human and temperature sensitivity. Consequently, a conventional whole-segment phylogenetic analysis might not disclose the many clinically and epidemiologically relevant sequence alterations, because the connections between particular specific phenotypic changes and their underlying genotypic variations might be masked with the intricate global effects of evolutionary selection on the whole viral genome. To deal with these constraints, we've developed a novel way of analyzing the effects of sequence variation on organism phenotypes known as the sequence feature variation form (SFVT) strategy, wherein mixtures of amino acid positions are described as distinct sequence attributes (SFs) according to structural and operational attributes. The amount of sequence variation is ascertained for every SF individually as a pair of version types (VTs) for the SF, which may subsequently be utilized for statistical evaluation of genotype-phenotype associations. The SFVT strategy was described for the institution from the setting of pancreatic.

Chapter - 1 Origin Of The Influenza Pandemic Of 1918-19

The sudden outbreak of the virus in 1918-19 was known as flu Pandemic. It was one of the most severe influenza outbreaks of the 20th century. In terms of absolute numbers of deaths, it was one of the most devastating pandemics in human history. Influenza is caused by a virus that's transmitted from person to person. An outbreak can happen from which the population has no immunity if a new strain of flu virus emerges. The flu pandemic of 1918-19 affected populations to a huge proportion. An influenza virus, known as flu type A subtype H1N1, is currently proven to have become the origin of the intense mortality of the outbreak, which led to an estimated 25 million deaths, even though some researchers have estimated it triggered as many as 40-50 million deaths. The pandemic occurred in 3 waves. The first seemingly originated in ancient March 1918, during World War I. Though it remains unclear at which the virus first surfaced, it rapidly spread through Western Europe, and by July it had spread to Poland. The initial wave of flu was mild. However, a kind of disorder had been known to be caused by it, and this type appeared in August 1918. Pneumonia developed after the initial indications of this influenza. As an instance, at Camp Devens, Massachusetts, U.S., six days after the first case of flu was reported, that there were 6,674 instances. The next wave of the pandemic happened in the next winter, and from the spring that the virus had run its program. In both waves roughly half of the deaths were among 20-40-year-olds, an odd mortality era pattern for flu. Outbreaks of this influenza occurred in almost every inhabited part of the world, first in vents, then dispersing from city to city across the primary transport routes. India is thought to have endured at 12.5 million deaths throughout the pandemic, and also the disease attained distant islands in the South Pacific, including New Zealand and Samoa. Roughly 550,000 people died. Most deaths happened during the third and second waves. Outbreaks of flu happened with virulence in the 1920s.

Epidemic

The epidemic is an incident of disorder that's temporarily high. If the incidence of an epidemic occurs over a large geographical area (e.g., globally), it is known as a pandemic. The rise and fall in the outbreak prevalence of infectious illness are likely to be occurred by the transport of an effective dose of the infectious agent from an infected person to a vulnerable person. Following an outbreak has escalated, the affected server population includes a sufficiently small percentage of susceptible people that reintroduction of this disease won't lead to a new outbreak. Considering that the parasite population can't replicate itself in this kind of bunch population, the host population as a whole is resistant to the epidemic disease, a phenomenon termed herd resistance. After an outbreak, the host population will revert into a state of susceptibility due to (1) the corrosion of human resistance; (2) the elimination of resistant people bypassing, and (3) the influx of vulnerable people by birth. With the years the people as a whole become more vulnerable. The time elapsing between outbreak peaks differs from another and is changeable. From the late 20th century that the definition of the outbreak was extended to include outbreaks of any chronic disease or illness (e.g., cardiovascular disease or obesity). The expression outbreak can be earmarked for illness among human beings; an epidemic of illness among animals aside from man is termed as epizootic.

Influenza

This is also known as a serious viral, grippe, or flu. This disease of the upper or lower respiratory tract is indicated by fever, chills, and a generalized feeling of pain and weakness in the muscles, as well as varying levels of soreness at the head and gut.

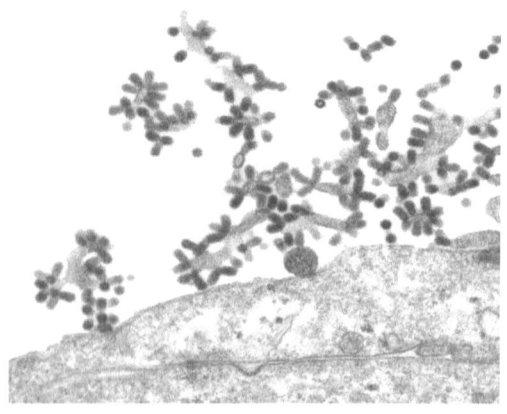

A Sequence Of Influenza Infection

This is any of the numerous sources of influenza viruses from the family Orthomyxoviridae (a group of RNA viruses). Flu viruses have been categorized as types A, B, C, D. These significant types normally produce similar symptoms but are unrelated antigenically, in order that infection with one type confers no resistance against the others. The A viruses trigger the excellent flu epidemics, along with the B germs trigger smaller localized outbreaks. C viruses cause a mild disease. Influenza D viruses aren't known to infect people and have been discovered only in cows. Influenza viruses are classified into subtypes, and subtypes of influenza A and the two influenza B are split into breeds. Subtypes of influenza A are distinguished mainly on the basis of two surface antigens (foreign proteins) --hemagglutinin (H) and neuraminidase (N). Cases of flu subtypes comprise H1N1, H5N1, and H3N2. Strains of influenza strains and B of flu subtypes are further distinguished by variations in the molecular arrangement.

Evolution And Virulence Of Influenza Infection

Between outbreaks, the pandemics viruses undergo continuously, rapid development (a procedure called antigenic drift), which can be powered by mutations in the genes encoding antigen proteins. Gradually, the viruses experience significant evolutionary change by obtaining a new genome section from a different flu virus (antigenic shift), effectively turning into a new subtype. Animals facilitate evolution. If a pig is concurrently infected with distinct influenza viruses, like human, swine, and avian strains, genetic reassortment could happen. This procedure contributes to new strains of influenza A. Recently surfaced flu viruses are inclined to be initially highly infectious and infectious in humans due to the fact that they have novel antigens to the body does not have any ready immune defense (i.e., present antibodies). After an important percentage of people develop resistance through the creation of antibodies capable of preventing the brand-new virus, the infectiousness and virulence of this virus decrease. Although outbreaks of flu viruses are usually most deadly to immature children and the elderly, the casualty rate in people between ages 20 and 40 is occasionally high, though the patients get therapy. This phenomenon is thought to be attributed to the hyper-reaction of their immune system to new strains of the flu virus. Response results in the overproduction of inflammatory chemicals called cytokines. The discharge of excessive quantities of these molecules induces inflammation that is acute. People whose immune systems aren't fully developed (like babies) or are diminished (like the older) can't create such a deadly immune reaction.

Pandemics And Epidemics

Influenza pandemics are estimated to occur on an average of every 50 decades. Epidemics might happen and the flu appears annually sometimes. A pandemic can happen within a matter of weeks, as soon as influenza a virus undergoes an antigenic change. The flu pandemic of 1918-19, the very damaging flu outbreak in history and among the most acute disease pandemics that ever struck, was due to a subtype of influenza called H1N1. In this event, an estimated 25 million individuals world-wide died of this so-called Spanish influenza, which was widely reported in Spain but originated from Kansas, U.S.

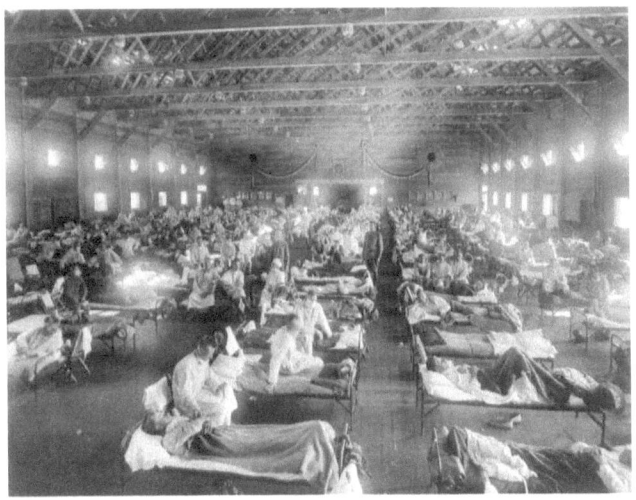

Pandemics of flu have been intense. For example, influenza A subtype H2N2, or the 1957 influenza pandemic, seemingly started in East Asia early in 1957, and by midyear it had circled the world. The outbreak continued to a pandemic amount until roughly the middle of 1958 and caused an estimated 1 million to 2 million deaths globally. Following 10 decades of development that generated yearly epidemics, the 1957 flu vanished in 1968, just to be replaced with a new influenza A subtype, H3N2. This virus is in circulation. The influenza outbreak of 1968 has been the third-largest flu pandemic of the 20th century also led to an estimated 1 million to four million deaths. In 1997 a kind of avian flu, or bird flu, virus awakened among domesticated poultry in Hong Kong, then infected a few individuals, killing a number of them. The exact same virus, H5N1, reappeared in one of the poultry flocks in Southeast Asia through the winter of 2003-04, infecting some individuals fatally. It hasoccasionally reappeared, mostly in wild birds, domestic poultry, and people. A lot of subtypes of bird influenza viruses have been known, such as H7N2, H7N3, and H9N2.

An epidemic of a strain of H1N1 happened in 2009. Initially called swine flu since the virus has been supposed to have been transmitted to humans from pigs; the disease initially broke out in Mexico and subsequently dispersed to the USA. The H1N1 virus that caused the epidemic was found to own genetic material from human, avian, and 2 distinct swine flu viruses. The 2009 H1N1 epidemic was not as fatal as the pandemic of 1918-19. The virus has been spread and highly infectious. The pandemic possibility of this new H1N1 virus has been made apparent to the global community from the World Health Organization (WHO), which broadcasted degree 5 pandemic alerts on April 29, 2009. This prompted the implementation of reduction processes in nations, to treatment centers. Despite all these steps, the virus continued to spread. On June 11, 2009, after an increase in cases in Chile, Australia, and the UK, WHO increased the H1N1 alert level from 5 to 6, which means that the outbreak was formally announced a pandemic. From 2010 individuals in over 209 nations had been affected. It was the first influenza pandemic of the 21st century. In the US, the elevated levels of disease observed through the 2009 pandemic weren't detected again until 2018. Studies have suggested that all the four historical flu pandemics was preceded by a La Niña occasion:a shift in global climate conditions related to cool sea surface temperatures from the Pacific Ocean that some scientists speculate could have shifted the migratory patterns of birds, potentially increasing their interactions with domestic animals and empowering hereditary variety and the growth of new pandemic strains of flu viruses.

Influenza Pandemic Preparedness

Because flu epidemics and pandemics can devastate areas of the planet quickly, WHO monitors flu disease activity on a worldwide scale. This observation is helpful for collecting information that may be employed to prepare vaccines and that may be disseminated to health centers in states where seasonal flu outbreaks will likely happen. Tracking by WHO pandemics plays a significant part in preventing and preparing for epidemics. In case a flu virus appears, WHO adheres to its pandemic preparedness program. This strategy contains six phases of pandemic alert. Phases 1-3, which are the phases in preparedness, are all made to stop or contain outbreaks that were modest. In these early stages, isolated incidences of both animal-to-human transmissions of a flu virus have been detected and supply warning signals that a virus has pandemic potential. Little outbreaks of the disorder may occur resulting, from instances of transmission. Stage 3 signs to states that are affected by the execution of attempts are required to protect against a pandemic. Phases 5 and 4 have been characterized in mitigating the outbreak by urgency. Confirmed human-to-human viral transmission, together with the continual disease in human communities that spread in order that disease transmission between individuals happened in just two states, suggests that a pandemic is imminent. Stage 6 is characterized by illness and transmission of the virus between people. Influenza pandemics happen in waves. Consequently, when illness activity decreases a stage, it might be accompanied by another phase of a high incidence of disease. Because of this, flu pandemics may persist for a period of weeks.

Transmission And Migraines

People of all ages may get affected; however, the prevalence of this disease is one of the adults and kids. Illness is transmitted from person to person in this way as inhalation of droplets leading to coughing and coughing. Since the virus particles gain entry, they ruin and attack the epithelial cells, which line the respiratory tract, bronchial tubes, and trachea. The incubation period of the illness is one or two days, and the symptoms are sudden, with abrupt and different distress, fatigue, and muscular aches. The temperature rises quickly to 38-40 °C (101-104 °F). Acute aches throughout the body and a headache are accompanied by a feeling of rawness in the throat or aggravation. A few times the fever starts to drop, and the individual starts to recover. Feelings of fatigue may be notable and accompany symptoms like coughing and nasal discharge. Complications like pneumonia or pneumonia may occur among individuals and may cause death.

Treatment And Prevention

The antiviral medications rimantadine and amantadine have consequences on instances of influenza between this type A virus. But immunity to these agents has already been detected, thereby decreasing their efficacy. A more recent category of medication, the neuraminidase inhibitors, including oseltamivir (Tamiflu) and zanamivir (Relenza), was released in the late 1990s; those drugs inhibit both the influenza A and B viruses. Aside from this, an intake of fluids, bed rest, and using analgesics is suggested. It's advised as treatment of diseases with aspirin is associated with Reye syndrome, that children and teenagers with the flu not to be given aspirin. Injection of a vaccine may bolster defense against the flu. These germs are produced in chick embryos; preparations that were regular incorporate a number of those a subtypes and the type B flu virus. Security from 1 vaccination lasts annually, and vaccination may be recommended for those people that are vulnerable to flu or whose condition could lead to complications. But immunization in healthy individuals is advised. Advances in the comprehension of influenza and flu technologies enabled the growth of a universal flu vaccine effective at protecting people against a range of flu subtypes.

To be able to prevent bird influenza viruses that are

human-infecting out of mutating into more harmful subtypes, public health authorities attempt to restrict the viral "reservoir" in which antigenic change may happen by ordering the destruction of infected poultry flocks.

Pandemic

Pandemic is connected to the geographical area and it might end up affecting a considerable percentage of the planet's inhabitants over the course of many months. Pandemics originate from epidemics, that can be outbreaks of disease restricted to a single portion, like a nation. To ensure that a post-period might be accompanied by another phase of high disease incidence, particularly those involving flu, pandemics happen in waves. Diseases like flu can spread in a matter of days. Numerous factors facilitate the spread of illness, such as an elevated amount of human-to-human transmission of this illness infectiousness of this representative, and way of transport. Diseases that arise in animals cause the vast majority. Therefore, when a new infectious agent or disorder occurs in creatures, surveillance organizations situated within impacted regions are responsible for alerting the World Health Organization (WHO) and also for carefully tracking the behavior of this infectious agent and also the action and spread of this illness. WHO monitors disease action on a worldwide scale by means of a network of surveillance centers found in nations. In the case of flu, WHO has arranged a pandemic preparedness plan that consists of six phases of pandemic alert, summarized as follows:

• Stage 1: the smallest level of pandemic alert; suggests an influenza virus, possibly just appeared or formerly present, is circulating among creatures. The chance of transmission to humans is reduced.

• Stage 2: isolated incidences of animal-to-human

transmission of this virus have been detected, suggesting that the virus has pandemic potential.

•   Stage 3: characterized by little outbreaks of disorder, normally resulting from several instances of animal-to-human transmission, even though limited capability for human-to-human transmission could be present.

•   Stage 4: supported human-to-human viral transmission which leads to sustained disease in human communities. At this point, containment of the virus is deemed hopeless but there is an inevitable pandemic. The implementation of management methods to prevent additional spread is highlighted in areas of the planet.

•   Stage 5: indicated with human-to-human disease transmission in just two states, signaling that a pandemic is imminent and that supply of stockpiled drugs and implementation of approaches to control the disorder has to be carried out with urgency.

•   Stage 6: characterized by sustained and widespread disease transmission among individuals.

When WHO updates a pandemic alert from level 4 to level 5, it functions as a sign to nations to execute the strategies that are suitable. Pandemics of diseases like cholera, plague, and flu have played a part in forming human cultures. Examples of important historic pandemics contain the plague outbreak of the Portuguese Empire in the 6th century CE; the Black Death, that originated in China and spread throughout Europe from the 14th century; along with the flu pandemic of 1918-19, that originated from the U.S. state of Kansas and spread into Europe, Asia, and islands in the South Pacific. Now several diseases happen on a worldwide scale persist in a high degree of incidence, though pandemics are characterized by their incidence on a length of time, and maybe transmitted between individuals. Such ailments represented in contemporary pandemics contain AIDS, caused by HIV (human immunodeficiency virus), which can be transmitted directly between individuals; and malaria, due to parasites in the genus Plasmodium, which can be transferred from one creature to another by mosquitoes, which feed on the blood of infected individuals.

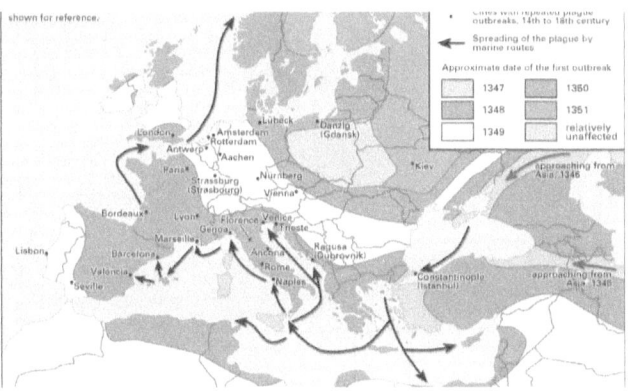

Influenza pandemics are anticipated to occur approximately every 50 decades, although the period in its occurrence has been shorter than that. After 191–9, you will find just two additional flu pandemics: the 1957 Asian flu and the 1968 Hong Kong influenza pandemic. Until about 1958, a pandemic arose that was responsible for over a million deaths. The influenza pandemic happened in 2009 when a subtype of virus spread across areas of the earth. Between March 2009 and mid-January 2010, H1N1 deaths were reported. In March 2020 an outbreak of a Novel coronavirus called severe acute respiratory syndrome coronavirus-2 (SARS-CoV2) was announced by WHO officials. Infection with SARS-CoV2 generated an illness called coronavirus disorder 2019 (COVID-19); the disease was characterized by cough, fever, and shortness of breath. The outbreak started at Wuhan, China in 2019, as soon as a patient with disabilities was admitted to a hospital. In the next few weeks, the number of individuals climbed in ratio, along with the spread of the Wuhan Disease into other areas of China. By 2020, COVID-19 had covered the USA and Europe by travelers. From the time the epidemic was announced, instances of COVID-19 had been discovered worldwide. There were confirmed cases and about 5,000 deaths.

Chapter - 2 The Origin And History Of Spanish Flu

This flu's source has been debated. The Claude Hannoun Pasteur Institute has posited that the virus originated in China, dispersed through troop moves, and from there, to Boston and Kansas, then to Brest, France. Here's a timeline of the Spanish Flu rallied around the globe.

April 1917 - the U.S. enters World War I with 378,000 guys in the armed forces, this can quickly swell to countless guys.

June 1917 - to raise the amount of men, there is a draft created. The military creates each home 25,000 to 55,000 guys, 32 training facilities.

March 1918 - That number increased five-fold a week later. Sporadic cases of the influenza start appearing elsewhere in the U.S., also in Europe and Asia.

April 1918 - that the mention of this influenza seems describing three deaths and 18 cases.

May 1918 - that the U.S. started shipping thousands upon thousands of troops to Europe. Due to the war, censors at Germany, England, France, and the U.S. were blocking news of this epidemic, leaving unbiased Spain to report the disorder. This is how it got the title, the "Spanish Flu." The virus spreads from Europe into North America, Asia, Africa, Brazil, islands in the South Pacific, as well as indigenous tribes living in the Arctic Circle.

September 1918 - another wave of this virus emerges, which has a higher fatality rate than the previous wave. It evolved in an Army facility, also in a Navy facility in Boston just outside the city.

This tide is responsible for the majority of the deaths in the virus, with 12,000 people dying from the U.S. through September. The New York City Board of Health required that cases of influenza be reported and patients are isolated, either in home or in a hospital. To get a Liberty Bonds parade, 200,000 people collect back in Philadelphia, and day's 635 cases of the flu are reported. Theaters, churches, and the town dictate schools were closed.

October 1918 - 195,000 Americans die of the flu in this month. There's a shortage of nurses since most are currently serving. The American Red Cross Chicago Chapter issues a call for volunteers to nurse the ill. Colleges and film theaters close, and public gatherings are prohibited by them. Legislation in Chicago drops by 43 percent. Is made to put away corpses and also a secondhand automobile maker requires packing crates to be utilized as coffins. San Francisco urges that face masks are worn by of its citizens out in people, and in NYC, shipbuilding is down by 40 percent because of absenteeism.

November 1918 - Soldiers are brought cases of the influenza, and back home by the conclusion of the war. Signals are placed by officials at Salt Lake City. In France, the armistice is signed on November 11, 1918, ending WWI. U.S. President Woodrow Wilson collapses after coming down with the flu.

January 1919 - a wave of the virus emerges, killing a lot people. Between January 1ˢᵗ and the fifth, 1,800 influenza cases that are new are experienced by San Francisco, and 101 people perish. New York City reports 706 cases and 67 deaths.

August 1919 - the Influenza pandemic comes to a conclusion because people who have been infected perished or developed resistance.

March 1997 - onMarch 21st, 1997, an article is published in Science Magazine. Researchers at the Armed Forces Institute of Pathology examined lung tissue obtained by a soldier that died in 1918 of this influenza. They conclude that although the influenza virus is exceptional, that, "The hemagglutinin receptor matches closest to swine flu viruses, demonstrating that this virus came to individuals through pigs."

February 2004 - Researchers at the Scripps Institute in La Jolla, California and in England's Medical Research Council conclude that the 1918 virus could have jumped directly from birds to people, bypassing dinosaurs entirely. This may explain the virulence of this disease.

October 2005 - Scientists in the Armed Forces Institute of Pathology order the whole genome of this virus by analyzing cells taken in the entire body of a flu sufferer whose body was preserved in permafrost because he had been buried in 1918.

Etymology

Despite its title, epidemiological and historic data can't identify the origin of the flu. The source of this "Spanish influenza" title comes out of the pandemic's spread to Spain from France in November 1918. Spain wasn't involved having stayed neutral, and hadn't enforced censorship during wartime. Newspapers were free to report the epidemic's effects, like the grave illness of King Alfonso XIII, and such widely-spread stories generated a false belief. Almost a century after the influenza struck in 1918--1920, the World Health Oganization (WHO) called on scientists, national governments and the press to follow best practices in discovering fresh human infectious diseases to minimize unnecessary adverse consequences on states, economies and individuals. More modern terms with this virus comprise the "1918 flu pandemic," the"1918 influenza pandemic," or variants of them.

Hypotheses Concerning The Origin

British Troops In France

The UK troop hospital and staging camp at Étaples in Virologist John Oxford has speculated France as being in the middle of the flu. His analysis found that with high mortality, which caused symptoms like the flu, the Étaples camp had been struck by the beginning of a disease at 1916. Based on Oxford, a similar outbreak occurred in March 1917 at military barracks at Alders, and military pathologists afterwards realized these premature outbreaks were the exact same disorder as the 1918 influenza. Hospital and the camp were perfect sites for dispersing the virus. The hospital treated 100,000 soldiers, victims of warfare, and chemical attacks. It was home to a piggery, and poultry had been brought in for food supplies in villages. His group and oxford declared that a metric virus, sailed to pigs and harbored in critters, mutated. A report printed in 2016 at the Journal of the Chinese Medical Association discovered signs that the 1918 virus was circulating in the European armies for months and maybe years prior to the 1918 pandemic.

United States

There have been announcements that the outbreak originated in the United States. Historian Alfred W. Crosby said in 2003 that the influenza originated in Kansas, and popular writer John M. Barry explained a January 1918 outbreak in Haskell County, Kansas as the point of origin from his 2004 article. A 2018 analysis of tissue slides and clinical reports directed by evolutionary research scientist Michael Worobec discovered evidence contrary to the disorder arising out of Kansas, as these instances had fewer deaths when compared with the situation in NYC at precisely the exact same period of time. The study failed to find signs; though it wasn't conclusive, the virus had a source. Additionally, the haemagglutinin glycoproteins of the virus imply that it had been around long until 1918 along with another research imply that the reassortment of the H1N1 virus probably occurred in roughly 1915.

China

Among the regions of the world apparently influenced from the 1918 influenza pandemic was China, in which there might have been a relatively mild flu season in 1918 (though this is disputed because of absence of information throughout the Warlord Period of China, visit Around the world). Studies have reported that there were deaths in comparison to other areas of earth. This has caused speculation that the 1918 influenza pandemic originated in China. Rates of influenza mortality in China in 1918 and the flu season might be clarified by the population acquired immunity to the influenza virus. In 1993, the expert for the Pasteur Institute about the 1918 flu, Claude Hannoun, claimed the virus was likely to have come from China. It then mutated in the USA near Boston and from there spread to Brest, France, Europe's battlefields, Europe, and the planet with Allied soldiers and sailors as the main disseminators. In 2014, historian Mark Humphries contended the mobilization of all laborers to operate behind the French and British lines could have been the origin of the pandemic. Humphries, of the Memorial University of Newfoundland in St. John's, based his decisions on recently unearthed records. He discovered evidence was identified by health officials equal to the flu. A report printed in 2016 at the Journal of the Chinese Medical Association found no signs that the 1918 virus had been imported to Europe through Chinese and Southeast Asian soldiers and employees, butinstead found signs of its flow in Europe prior to the pandemic. The 2016 study indicated that the very low flu mortality rate (an estimated 1/1000) found one of the Chinese and Southeast Asian employees in Europe meant the deadly 1918 flu pandemic couldn't have originated from these employees. A 2018 analysis of tissue slides and clinical reports directed by evolutionary research scientist Michael Worobey discovered evidence contrary to the disease being distributed by Chinese employees, noting that employees entered Europe via other avenues, which didn't lead to detectable spread, making them unlikely to have been the original hosts.

Additional

Hannoun considered different hypotheses of source, like Spain, Kansas, and Brest, as potential, but not probable. Political scientist Andrew Price-Smith published information in the archives in Austria, 1917.

Spread

When an infected person sneezes or coughs, million virus particles can disperse to people nearby. Troop movements of World War I and close quarters hastened both transmissions, and likely the pandemic and mutation that were augmented. The lethality of the virus might have increased. Some speculate that the soldiers' immune systems were weakened, in addition to by malnourishment. An element in the occurrence of the flu was raised journey. Modern transport systems made it much easier for sailors, soldiers, and even travelers to spread the illness. The following was refusal and lies by authorities.

The disorder was observed in Haskell County, Kansas, in January 1918, prompting local physician Loring Miner to frighten that the US Public Health Service's educational diary. About 4 March 1918, firm cook Albert Gitchell, from Haskell County, reported ill at Fort Riley, a US military facility that at the time had been training American troops during World War I, making him the first recorded victim of the influenza. In days, guys in the camp had reported ill. About 11 Queens had been conquered by the virus. Everyone was struggling to take steps to counter it but their actions were criticized. In August 1918, a more virulent strain appeared concurrently in Brest, France; at Freetown, Sierra Leone; and at the U.S., in September, in the Boston Navy Yard and Camp Devens (later renamed Fort Devens), roughly 30 kilometers west of Boston. Other U.S. military websites were shortly affected, as were soldiers being hauled to Europe. By returning soldiers, the influenza carried there.

Mortality

Around The World

The influenza effected about a quarter of the planet's inhabitants. Estimates as to how many infected individuals died vary considerably, but the influenza was not regarded as among the deadliest pandemics. A quote from 1991 claims that the virus killed between 25 and 39 million individuals. A 2005 estimate put the death toll in 50 million (less than 3 percent of the worldwide population), and maybe as large as 100 million (greater than 5 percent). However, a reassessment at 2018 estimated the total to be approximately 17 million, although this was contested. With a world population of 1.8 to 1.9 billion, these estimates correspond between 1 and 6% of the populace. This influenza killed more people than The Black Death, that lasted longer, murdered a proportion of the world's smaller inhabitants. The illness killed in regions of the planet. A few 12-17 million people died roughly 5 percent of the populace, in India. The death toll in India's British-ruled districts was 13.88 million. Arnold (2019) quotes at least 12 million deceased. Estimates for its death toll in China have varied, which reflects the absence of group of health data. The first quote of this Chinese death toll has been created in 1991 by Patterson and Pyle, which estimated China needed a death toll of between 5 and 9 million. But studies as a result of faulty methodology criticized this 1991 analysis, and studies have released estimates of a mortality rate in China. As an example, Iijima in 1998 estimates that the death toll in China to be between 1 and 1.28 million according to information accessible Chinese port towns. Since, Wataru Iijima notes,' Pyle and Patterson within their research 'The 1918 Influenza Pandemic' attempted to gauge the amount of deaths as a whole from the flu in China. They contended between 4.0 and 9.5 million people died in China, yet this total was established purely on the premise that the passing rate there was 1.0--2.25 percent in 1918, since China was a bad nation very similar to Indonesia and India in which the mortality rate was of the purchase. Their analysis wasn't based on any statistical information. The lower estimates of the Chinese death toll derive from the minimal mortality rates, which were discovered in Chinese port towns (by way of instance, Hong Kong) and also on the premise that poor communications prevented the influenza from entering the inside of China. But some modern post and newspaper office reports, in addition to reports from missionary physicians, imply the influenza failed to penetrate the Chinese inside and that flu was awful in certain places in the countryside of China.

23 million people were affected; with at least deaths were reported by 390,000. From the Dutch East Indies (now Indonesia), 1.5 million were supposed to have expired among 30 million individuals. In Tahiti, 13 percent of the people died during a month. In the same way, in just two months, 22 percent of the populace of 38,000 died at Samoa. In New Zealand, the flu killed an estimated 6,400 Pakeha and 2,500 native Maori in fourteen days, together with Māori expiring at eight times the speed of Pakeha.

In Iran, the Mortality was quite high:

• According to a quote, 8 to 22 percent of the

population, or involving 902,400 and 2,431,000 expired.

In the U.S., roughly 28 percent of the Populace of 105 million became infected, and 500,000 to 850,000 expired (0.48 to 0.81 percentage of the populace). Native American tribes were hard hit. There have been deaths among Americans. Alaskan village communities and whole Inuit expired in Alaska. 50,000 expired. In Britain, as many as in France, Alves Back in Brazil, over 400,000. In Ghana, at least 100,000 individuals were killed by the flu epidemic. Tafari Makonnen (the near future Haile Selassie, Emperor of Ethiopia) was among those earliest Ethiopians who contracted flu but lived. Many of the subjects didn't; quotes for deaths from the capital city include even higher or even 5,000 to 10,000. In British Somaliland, 1 official estimated that 7 percent of the population died. This death toll caused from an infection rate of the seriousness of these symptoms and also around 50%, suspected to be brought on by storms. Symptoms in 1918 were uncommon causing flu. 1 contributor wrote, "Among the most notable of these complications was hemorrhage from mucous membranes, particularly from the nose, stomach, and intestine. Bleeding from the ears and petechial hemorrhages in skin also happened". The vast majority of deaths have been a secondary disease, from pneumonia. By inducing hemorrhages and edema in the 15, the virus murdered people.

Patterns Of Fatality

Adults were killed by the pandemic. Back in 1918–1919, 99 percent of pandemic flu deaths from the U.S. happened in people under 65, and almost half of deaths were in

29

young adults 20 to 40 years old. The mortality rate among people under 65 had diminished six-fold but 92 percent of deaths occurred in people. Because the flu is generally deadly to individuals, like infants under age 2 and the immune compromised, this is uncommon. Back in 1918, older adults might have experienced partial protection brought on by exposure to the 1889-1890 influenza pandemic, called the "Russian flu." Based on historian John M. Barry, the most exposed of– "those probably, of the very likely", to perish -- were pregnant ladies. He reported in thirteen researches of women in the pandemic, the death rate ranged from 23 to 71 percent. Of those pregnant women who lived childbirth, over one-quarter (26 percent) dropped the kid. The other oddity was that the epidemic was prevalent at the summer and fall (from the Northern Hemisphere); flu is generally worse in the winter. Contemporary research has proven that the virus to be especially deadly because it activates a cytokine storm (overreaction of the body's immune system), which ravages the more powerful immune system of young adults. The virus was retrieved by 1 set of investigators in the bodies of creatures that were transfected and victims with it. The creatures suffered progressive respiratory failure and passing. Whereas the poorer reactions of adults and kids resulted in deaths, the immune reactions of adults have been postulated to have shattered the entire body. By consolidation, mortality has been mostly in scenarios. Cases comprised neural involvement that led sometimes to mental disorders, and bacterial infections. Some deaths were the result of malnourishment. A research conducted employed a mechanistic modeling approach to examine the 3 waves of the 1918 flu pandemic. They analyzed the elements that underlie variability in their significance and patterns to patterns of morbidity and mortality. Their analysis indicates that the explanation is provided by variations in transmission speed, and also the variation is inside plausible values. Another analysis by The et al. (2013) employed a simple epidemic model comprising three variables to infer the reason for the 3 waves of the 1918 flu pandemic. These variables were closure and college opening, temperature changes during the outbreak, and individual modifications in response to this outbreak. The consequences were shown by behavioral reactions, although their modeling results demonstrated that all three variables are significant. A 2020 analysis found that US towns, which implemented extensive and early non-medical measures (quarantine etc.) endured no further adverse financial consequences because of implementing those steps, compared to cities that implemented steps late or in any way.

Deadly Second Tide

The wave of the 1918 pandemic was more deadly compared to first. The wave had resembled flu epidemics; people most in danger were older and the ill, whereas fitter people recovered. From August, once the second wave started in Sierra Leone France and the USA, the virus had mutated into a form. October 1918 was the month with the maximum fatality rate of the pandemic in its entirety. This seriousness was credited to the conditions of the First World War. In life, a strain is favored by natural selection. From the trench's selection was reversed. Where they had been soldiers with a strain remained, while the ill were sent to area hospitals to trains, dispersing the more deadly virus. The second wave started, and the entire world was spread across by the influenza. Thus, during modern pandemics, health officials listen once the virus reaches areas with societal upheaval (searching for deadlier strains of this virus). The simple fact that the majority of people who recovered from ailments that were first-wave had become immune revealed that it has to have been the strain of influenza. This was dramatically exemplified in Copenhagen, which escaped using a joint mortality rate of just 0.29percent (0.02 percent in the initial wave and 0.27 percent in the next wave) due to vulnerability to the less-lethal first tide. For the remaining portion of the populace, the next wave was much more mortal; the individuals that were most exposed were those such as the soldiers in the trenches -- adults that were fit and youthful.

Devastated Communities

Mass graves were dug by steam shovel and bodies buried without coffins in many areas. Pacific island lands were hit hard. The pandemic reached them from New Zealand, which had been slow to execute measures to stop from leaving its vents, boats, like the SS Talune, taking the flu. By New Zealand, the influenza attained Tonga (murdering 8 percent of the populace), Nauru (16 percent), and Fiji (5 percent, 9,000 individuals). Worst was Western Samoa German Samoa that was inhabited by New Zealand in 1914. 90 percent of the population was infected; 22 percent of women 30 percent of men, and 10 percent of kids died. By comparison, the flu was prevented by Governor John Martin Poyer by means of a blockade from reaching American Samoa. The disease spread quickest through the social groups among the peoples, due to the habit of collecting heritage from chiefs in their deathbed's community elders were infected through this procedure. In New Zealand, 8,573 deaths have been attributed to the 1918 pandemic flu, leading to an entire population fatality rate of 0.7 percent. Māori were 8 to 10 times less likely to die as Pakeha, due to the comparative poverty, more crowded home, rural inhabitants and lesser resistance to illness. In 1918, the influenza accounted for 10 percent of the deaths in Ireland.

Less-Affected Places

China might have undergone a mild flu season in 1918 in comparison to other regions of the planet. There was no group of health data in the nation at the moment, and a few reports out of its inside indicate that mortality rates from flu were greater in at least a few places in China. At the minimum, there's minimal proof that the influenza affected China as a whole in contrast to other nations on earth. Though records from the inside of China are missing, there was information listed in, like Harbin, Canton, Peking, Hong Kong and Shanghai. The Chinese Maritime Customs Service that has been staffed by foreigners, like the British, French, and other colonial officials in China gathered this information. As a complete, low mortality rates are shown by true data from the port towns of China in comparison to other towns in Asia. For instance, the British government at Hong Kong and Canton reported a mortality rate from flu at a speed of 0.25 and 0.32 percent, considerably lower than the reported mortality rate of different cities in Asia, for example Calcutta or Bombay, at which flu was a lot more catastrophic. From Shanghai's city -- that had a population of more than 2 million that there were only 266 deaths from flu among the people in 1918. If extrapolated in the extensive data listed from Chinese towns, the proposed mortality rate from flu in China as a whole in 1918 was probably lower than 1 percent -- considerably lower than the world average (that was approximately 3--5 percent). By comparison, Japan and Taiwan had reported a mortality rate from flu around 0.45% and 0.69% respectively, greater than the mortality rate accumulated from statistics in Chinese port cities, including Hong Kong (0.25 percent), Canton (0.32 percent), and Shanghai. Back in Japan, 257,363 deaths have been attributed to the flu by July 1919, providing an estimated 0.4 percent mortality rate, which was considerably lower than almost all other Asian nations for which data are readily available. When the pandemic struck, the authorities restricted sea traveling to and from.

In American Samoa, the Pacific and the colony of New Caledonia succeeded in preventing a single death through quarantines. Almost 12,000 expired. From the conclusion of the island of Marajó, the pandemic in Brazil's Amazon River Delta hadn't reported an outbreak. No deaths were reported by Saint Helena. The passing although the epidemiologists that toll in Russia was estimated at 450,000. If it is right, Russia lost percent of its inhabitants -- the lowest mortality in Asia. This is considered by another study. The infrastructure of life had broken down

Death toll was closer to 2 percent, or 2.7 million people.

Aspirin Poisoning

In 2009, a paper printed in the journal Clinical Infectious Karen Starko suggested that aspirin poisoning contributed to the deaths. She based that on the reported symptoms of people dying from the flu, as mentioned from the post mortem reports still accessible, as well as the timing of this large "departure spike" in October 1918. This happened shortly after the Surgeon General of the U.S. Army, along with the Journal of the American Medical Association, both advocated quite massive doses of 2 to 31 grams of aspirin daily as part of therapy. These amounts created hyperventilation in lung edema in 3 percent of patients, in addition to 33 percent of patients. Starko additionally notes that lots of premature deaths demonstrated "moist," occasionally hemorrhagic lungs, whereas late deaths revealed bacterial pneumonia. She indicates that the tide of aspirin poisonings was the result of a "perfect storm" of events: Bayer's patent on aspirin died, so many companies rushed in to earn a gain and significantly increased the source; this collaborated with the Spanish influenza; and the indications of aspirin poisoning weren't known at the moment. For example, for its high mortality rate, this theory was contested in a letter to the journal printed in April 2010 by Andrew Noymer and Daisy Carreon of the University of California, Irvine, and Niall Johnson of the Australian Commission on Safety and Quality in Healthcare. They contested the applicability of this aspirin concept, given that the high mortality rate in which there was no or little access to aspirin in the moment, in contrast to the death rate in areas. They reasoned that "the salicylate aspirin poisoning theory was hard to maintain as the most important explanation for the unusual virulence of the 1918-1919 flu pandemic." In reaction, Starko stated there was scientific evidence of aspirin usage in India and contended that if aspirin over-prescription hadn't contributed to the elevated Indian mortality rate, it might still happen to be a factor for elevated rates in locations where other exacerbating factors found in India played a function.

End Of The Pandemic

Following the deadly wave struck instances that are fresh, in 1918 dropped from the wave. By way of instance, 4,597 people died in the week ending 16 October, but from town, the flu had vanished by 11 November. One explanation for the rapid decrease from the lethality of this disease is that physicians became effective in prevention and therapy of their pneumonia that developed following the sufferers that contracted the virus. Some cases that are mortal did last into March 1919. Another theory maintains that the 1918 virus mutated into a strain. This is a frequent phenomenon with flu viruses: there's a trend for pathogenic viruses to be less deadly with time, as the hosts of dangerous breeds have a tendency to expire (see also "Deadly Second Wave", above).

Long-Term Consequences

That was discovered by a 2006 research from the Journal of Political Economy "cohorts in utero" during the pandemic demonstrated reduced educational attainment, improved degrees of physical handicap, lower earnings, lower socioeconomic status, and greater transfer payments received in comparison to other birth cohorts. A 2018 research discovered that the pandemic decreased educational attainment in populations. The flu was connected from the 1920s to the epidemic of encephalitis lethargica.

Chapter - 3 What's Spanish Flu?

This influenza is also called the 1918 influenza pandemic, or the deadly flu. Lasting from January 1918 500 million people -- roughly a third of the planet's population – were infected by it. The death toll was estimated to have been everywhere from as large as 100 million, and 17 million to 50 million, which makes it among the deadliest pandemics in history. World War I censored diminished reports of mortality and illness in the USA, the UK, France, and Germany to preserve sanity. Newspapers were free to report the epidemic's effects in neutral Spain, like the grave illness of King Alfonso XIII, and such stories generated a false belief of Spain as particularly hard hit. This gave rise. Ancient and epidemiological data are insufficient to identify with certainty that the pandemics geographical source, with varying perspectives regarding its place. Most flu outbreaks kill the very young and the very old, using a greater survival rate for all those in between, but the Spanish influenza pandemic led to a greater than expected mortality rate for adults. Researchers provide several explanations for its high mortality rate of the 1918 flu pandemic. Some investigations have demonstrated the virus to be especially deadly because it activates a cytokine storm, which ravages the more powerful immune system of young adults. By comparison, a 2007 analysis of health care journals in the length of the pandemic discovered that the viral disease was not any more competitive than previous flu strains. Rather, hygiene, overcrowded spas and hospitals, and malnourishment encouraged infection. This infection was deadly to all victims. The Spanish influenza was the first of 2 pandemics caused by the flu virus; the next was that influenza in 2009.

What's The Flu?

Influenza, or flu, is a virus that attacks the respiratory system. The influenza virus is extremely infectious: If an infected person coughs, sneezes or talks, respiratory droplets are created and transmitted to the atmosphere, and may be inhaled by anyone near. Furthermore, someone who rolls something with the entire virus onto it and then touches their mouth, nose, or eyes may get infected. Flu outbreaks occur annually and change in severity, depending in part on which sort of virus is spreading. (Flu viruses can quickly mutate.)

Spanish Influenza: The Virus That Changed The World

A disorder started to sweep a deadly virus that infected a third of the planet's inhabitants and left upwards of 50 million dead. Laura Spinney investigated the devastating effect of the Spanish influenza pandemic and how it contrasted the Coronavirus disaster on 28 September 1918. A Spanish paper gave its viewers a brief lesson on flu. "The representative responsible for this disease, it is your Pfeiffer's bacillus, which is very tiny and observable only by way of a microscope." The explanation was because the entire world was in the grasp of their very barbarous influenza pandemic on record -- but it was wrong: influenza is caused by a virus. The concept that influenza was caused by a bacillus or Illness was approved by the most distinguished scientists of their day, who'd find themselves almost completely helpless in the face of the scourge.

Just How Many People Died From The Spanish Flu?

Spanish influenza was among the deadliest disasters in history. It lasted for 2 decades -- between the earliest documented instance in March 1918 and the past in March 1920, an estimated 50 million people died, although some experts indicate that the total could have been double. Even the 'Spanish flu' murdered during the First World War, maybe more than the Second World War.

How Can Spanish Influenza Compare To

Coronavirus?Laura Spinney told me "You may have observed a figure floating about of a case fatality rate of 3.4 percent, which describes the ratio of individuals who capture the COVID-19 disease who go to die of it. The amount that is frequently quoted for its Spanish Flu, as an instance, the case fatality rate is 2.5percent but it is a very, very, very controversial figure since the amounts are so obscure. I mean we believe that probably 50 million people died but there wasn't any kind of reliable test in the time so that we cannot be convinced about that which only cries all of the numbers out." So, it is really tough to create the historic comparisons, even in the event that you've got accurate data today, which we do not. Therefore, on either side of the equation, even if you prefer, it is a moving target. "We'd obviously love to get a vaccine from COVID-19 today but we do not and we might need to wait a year to 18 months because of that. They'd have no vaccine whatsoever in 1918. Or rather they did create molds but they were unworthy, pretty much, as they were basically pathogens against bacteria in the respiratory tract whereas, as we understand, influenza is a viral illness. So, regarding this, we're advanced compared to 1918. But we do not have that vaccine. We have anti-inflammatory medication for treating the ill and we have antibiotics that will be useful for treating the bacterial ailments that might lead to pneumonia sometimes, as they did in 1918, interestingly."

The pandemic struck in a vital juncture of comprehension of illness that is infectious. Well into the 19th century, epidemics were considered acts of God -- a belief that dated back into the Middle Ages. Originally, although compounds were observed in the 17th century, they were not connected with disorders. In the 1850s, the French biologist Louis Pasteur made the link between disorder and micro-organisms, and by a couple of microbiologist Robert Koch furthered notions of illness. 'Germ concept' was disseminated far and wide, replacing thoughts that were fatalistic. The 20th century, together with improvements in sanitation and hygiene, had made considerable inroads from the so-called 'audience' ailments that affected human communities, particularly those inhabiting the fantastic cities which had mushroomed in the aftermath of the industrial revolution. Through the 19th century many urbanites were dropped to diseases -- cholera, tuberculosis, and typhus, to mention three -- which cities had a continuous influx of peasants in the countryside to keep their numbers up. At last they had become self-explanatory.

Where Did The Spanish Flu Originate?

Some theories suggest it did not begin in Spain. We do not understand where it began, but we know it did not begin in Spain. The Spanish were, to a degree, stigmatized with this. Even though the trenches of the First World War are still a contender, there's also no means of being sure where Spanish Flu originated. The soldiers' immune system changed. It's believed before spreading at an alarming speed to Europe, the cases were the pandemic was known as 'Spanish Flu.' Censorship exaggerated the effects of the virus in Spain. While Britain, France, Germany, and the USA censored and limited early reports, newspapers in Spain -- as a neutral nation -- were liberated to communicate all of the dreadful details of this pandemic.

From 1918, faith in mathematics was low, and large scientists had adopted a swagger. Twenty years before, this had motivated the Irish playwright George Bernard Shaw to compose the physician's Dilemma, where an eminent physician, Sir Colenso Ridgeon -- a personality according to Sir Almroth Wright, who developed the typhoid vaccine -- plays god with his patients' destinies. Shaw was warning physicians against hubris; however, it required an epidemic of another 'audience' disorder -- flu -- to bring them home they understood. When scientists believed about 'germs' from the 20th century, they thought about germs. The virus was a novel theory; its capacity had infected tobacco plants and discovered the virus, found in 1892. Unlike germs, it had been too little to be viewed through an optical microscope. Without having really observed viruses, scientists mimicked their character. They had been veiled in mystery, and no one guessed that they might be the reason for the flu. Throughout the influenza pandemic -- the so-called 'Russian' flu, which started in 1889 -- a pupil of Koch's called Richard Pfeiffer promised to have identified. Pfeiffer's bacillus, as it had been known, can cause illness and does exist -- but it doesn't cause flu. During the 1918 pandemic, pathologists who cultivated bacterial colonies in the lung tissue of influenza victims discovered Pfeiffer's bacillus in certain, but not all of the civilizations, which puzzled them. To add to physicians' puzzlement, vaccines generated from the bacillus of Pfeiffer appeared to gain some patients. Actually, these experiments were successful against secondary bacterial diseases that caused pneumonia -- that the greatest cause of death in most instances -- but scientists did not understand that at the moment. They'd realize that it was a mistake.

Flu Season

In the USA, "flu season" normally runs from late Fall into spring. In a normal year, over 200,000 Americans are hospitalized for flu-related complications, and within the last 3 decades, there were several 3,000 to 49,000 flu-related U.S. deaths annually, according to the Centers for Disease Control and Prevention. Young kids, individuals over age 65, pregnant women, and individuals with particular medical conditions, like diabetes, asthma, or cardiovascular disease, face a greater chance of flu-related complications, such as pneumonia, sinus, ear infections and hepatitis. Influenza pandemic, like the one in 1918, happens when a particularly virulent new flu strain for which there is little if any immunity arises and spreads rapidly from person to person around the world.

Spanish Flu Symptoms

The initial wave of the 1918 pandemic happened in the spring and was mild. The ill, which underwent such common influenza symptoms like chills, fatigue, and fever, normally recovered after a few days, and also the number of reported deaths was reduced. The second wave of flu appeared in the autumn of that year with a vengeance. Victims died within days or hours of symptoms. By a couple of years, the average life expectancy in America dropped 1918, in 1 year.

What Led To The Spanish Flu?

It is unknown exactly where the specific breed of Flu that caused the pandemic originated. Nonetheless, the 1918 influenza was first detected in Europe, America, and regions of Asia before spreading to nearly every other portion of the world in a matter of weeks. Regardless of the fact that the 1918 influenza was not isolated to a location, it became famous around the world since Spanish influenza, Spain was struck hard by the illness and wasn't subject to the malevolent news blackouts that affected other European nations. (Spain's king, Alfonso XIII, allegedly contracted the flu) 1 odd aspect of the 1918 influenza was that it struck many formerly healthy, young individuals – a band generally resistant to this form of infectious disease – including lots of World War I servicemen. In reality, many more U.S. soldiers died from the 1918 influenza than were killed in the conflict during the war. Forty percent of the U.S. Navy was struck with the flu, while 36% of the Army became sick. Soldiers moving around the planet in crowded trains and ships helped to disperse the killer virus. Additional estimates run as large as 3% of the planet's inhabitants. The death toll attributed to the influenza is estimated at 20 million to 50 million sufferers globally. The numbers are not possible to understand because of a deficiency of health. What is known is that places were resistant to the 1918 influenza – to people of communities that were remote, victims ranged from residents of cities in America. Even President Woodrow Wilson allegedly contracted influenza in early 1919 while negotiating the Treaty of Versailles, which ended World War I.

Why Was The Spanish Flu Called Spanish?

The Spanish Flu didn't arise in Spain. Spain was a state with a press that covered the outbreak in Madrid in May from the beginning. Meanwhile, the Central Powers, as well as Allied nations, had censors who covered news of this influenza up to keep morale high. Since Spanish information resources were not the only ones reporting on influenza, many considered it originated there (the Spanish, meanwhile, considered the virus originated out of France and called it the "French Flu.")

Where Did The Spanish Flu Come From?

Scientists do not know for certain where the Flu originated. Concepts point to France, China, Britain, and also the USA, in which the earliest instance was reported on March 11, 1918, in Camp Funston at Fort Riley, Kansas. Some consider soldiers that were infected had spread the illness throughout the nation to army camps. In March 1918, the subsequent month soldiers led across the Atlantic and have been followed closely by 118,000 more.

First Instances Reported From The Deadly Spanish Influenza Pandemic

Before breakfast on the afternoon of March 4, Albert Mitchell of the U.S. Army reports on the hospital in Fort Riley, Kansas, whining of those cold-like symptoms of sore throat, pain, and fever. By comparison, over 100 of his fellow soldiers had reported symptoms that were similar, signaling what are thought to be the initial cases from the flu pandemic of 1918. Influenza would kill an estimated 20 million to 50 million people and 675,000 Americans across the world, proving to be a much more deadly force than the First World War. The outbreak of this disease has been accompanied by outbreaks in prisons and military camps in a variety of areas of the nation. The disease shortly traveled to Europe together with the American soldiers going to help the Allies in the battlefields of France (Back in March 1918 alone, 84,000 American soldiers led across the Atlantic; yet another 118,000 followed them another month). Influenza revealed no signs of abating when it came on another continent: 31,000 cases were reported in Great Britain in June. The disorder was soon dubbed Spanish influenza as a result of a shockingly higher number of deaths in Spain (some 8 million, it had been reported) following the first outbreak there in May 1918. No mercy was shown by influenza on each side of the trenches for combatants. The initial wave of the outbreak hit against German forces, in which they waged a closing offensive which could establish the results of the war. It had a substantial impact on the morale of their troops as the flu deepened losses, along with bad provisions depressing the spirits of guys in the III Infantry Division. The flu spread past the boundaries of Western Europe. The close of the summer had cases reported in Russia, North Africa, and India; New Zealand, Japan, the Philippines as well as China would fall victim. The Great War ended on November 11, but flu continued to wreak global havoc, flaring again in the U.S. within a more vicious wave together with the return of soldiers against the war and finally infecting an estimated 28 percent of the nation's population before it eventually petered out.

Fighting The Spanish Flu

Scientists and doctors were unsure after the 1918 flu strike what caused it or how to take care of it. There were drugs which treated the flu but no vaccines or antivirals. (The very first accredited flu vaccine emerged in America in the 1940s. By the next decade, vaccine makers could routinely create vaccines that would help restrain and protect against potential pandemics). Complicating matters was the fact that World War I had abandoned a lack of doctors and other health workers to portions of America. And of that available medical personnel from the U.S., many came back with the flu themselves. Hospitals in certain areas were bombarded with influenza patients who other buildings, private houses, and schools needed to be converted to hospitals, a few of which were staffed with students. Officials in certain areas imposed quarantines such as churches, schools, and theaters. People were advised also to remain inside and also to avoid shaking hands, libraries placed a block on regulations and financing books. According to the New York Times, throughout the ordeal, Boy Scouts in New York approached people they had seen spitting on the road and gave them cards which read: "You're in violation of this Sanitary Code."

Aspirin Poisoning And The Flu

Without treatment for the flu physicians, they believed it would relieve symptoms. For example: aspirin, which was trademarked by Bayer in 1899 – a patent which died in 1917, meaning fresh firms could create the medication during the Spanish Flu outbreak. Prior to the spike in deaths attributed to the Spanish Flu in 1918, the U.S. Surgeon General, Navy and also the Journal of the American Medical Association had recommended the use of aspirin. Medical professionals counseled patients to take around 30g every day. (For comparison's sake, the health consensus now is that doses over 4g is dangerous). Indicators of aspirin poisoning include the buildup of fluid in the lungs, or hyperventilation, and edema, and it believed that a number hastened or of those October deaths were caused by aspirin poisoning.

The Flu Takes Heavy Toll On Society

Influenza took countless lives; creating widows and orphans. Funeral parlors were filled with bodies as they began piling up. People needed to dig graves for their very own Relatives. The influenza was injurious to the market. From the United States, because many workers stated they were forced to shut down sick. Basic services like trash collection and mail delivery were hindered due to employees. There were farm employees to harvest plants. Even local and state health departments shut down for company, hampering attempts to supply and to chronicle the spread of the 1918 influenza People about it with responses.

The Way U.S. Cities Try To Stop The 1918 Flu Pandemic

A catastrophic tide of the Spanish Flu struck American beaches in the summer of 1918 and spread to various cities. With no vaccine or treatment program, it dropped to officials and mayors to improvise plans to protect the citizens. With pressure to appear patriotic at wartime and with a censored media downplaying the disease's spread, many made tragic decisions. The answer to Philadelphia was too little, too late. Dr. Wilmer Krusen, manager of Public Health and Charities for the town, insisted mounting deaths weren't the "Spanish flu," but instead the only influenza. The town moved with a Liberty Loan parade spreading the illness. More than 1,000 Philadelphians were lifeless. Only then did the city close saloons and theaters. From March 1919, their own lives had been lost by over 15,000 citizens of Philadelphia. St. Louis, Missouri, was distinct: Schools and film theaters closed and public parties were prohibited. As a result, the peak mortality rate in St. Louis was only one-eighth of Philadelphia's passing rate during the peak of the outbreak. Citizens at San Francisco were fined $5 when they had been caught with no masks and charged with disturbing the peace.

Spanish Flu Pandemic Ends

From the summer of 1919, the influenza pandemic came to an end; those who were infected either acquired resistance or expired. Nearly 90 decades after, in 2008, researchers announced they had found exactly what made the 1918 flu so fatal: A bunch of 3 genes allowed the virus to weaken a sufferer's bronchial tubes and lungs and clear the way for bacterial pneumonia. Too lethal, there were other flu pandemics since 1918. An influenza pandemic from 1957 to 1958 killed around two million people globally, such as some 70,000 people in America, along with also a pandemic from 1968 to 1969 killed approximately 1 million individuals, including some 34,000 Americans. Over 12,000 Americans expired during the H1N1 (or "swine flu") pandemic, which happened from 2009 to 2010. The novel coronavirus outbreak of 2020 is spreading around the globe as nations race to locate a remedy for COVID 19 and taxpayers refuge set up in an effort to prevent spreading the illness, which can be very deadly because most carriers are asymptomatic for times before recognizing they're infected. Every one of those modern-day pandemics brings renewed attention in and focus on the Spanish Flu, or "forgotten pandemic," so-named since its spread had been overshadowed by the deadliness of both WWI and coated by information blackouts and inadequate record-keeping.

Chapter - 4 Why Can It Be Known As 'Spanish Flu'?

Influenza had obtained its name as it had been thought to have originated from Bukhara in Uzbekistan (at the time, part of the Russian empire). The pandemic, which broke out almost 30 decades after will always be called the 'Spanish flu', although it did not begin in Spain. It washed across the entire world in three waves that, at the northern hemisphere, corresponded to some gentle wave in the spring of 1918, a deadly wave the subsequent fall, and reprisal from the first months of 1919, which was intermediate in virulence between both. The cases were listed at Camp Funston. Within six weeks that the illness had reached the trenches of the western front in France, however, it was only in May that influenza broke out in Spain. Contrary to the USA and France, Spain was neutral in the war; therefore it did not censor its own press. The first Spanish instances were reported in the papers, also since King Alfonso XIII, the prime minister, and many members of this cabinet were one of those early cases; the nation's plight was highly observable. People around the world thought that the disorder had rippled from Madrid -- a misconception encouraged by propagandists in these belligerent countries that knew they had contracted it before Spain. In the interest of maintaining morale high within their populations, they were pleased to change the blame. The title stuck. Understandably, Spaniards smarted at this calumny: they understood that they weren't accountable, and imagined the French of getting sent

52

influenza throughout the boundary, but they could not be convinced. They throw around for another tag, also found inspiration in an operetta performed in the capital Zarzuela Theatre -- a hugely popular reworking of the myth of Don Juan, with a catchy song called 'The Soldier of Naples'. The tricky disease became famous in Spain as the 'Naples Soldier.' Although the Spanish flu did not begin in Spain that nation did suffer very badly with it. From the early 20th century, influenza was regarded as a democratic disorder -- nobody was immune against it but, in the thick of this pandemic, it had been noticed that the disease struck. It 'favored' particular age classes: the very young and the older, but also a center cohort aged 20 to 40. It favored men to women, with the exclusion of pregnant ladies, who have been at especially large risk. This age and gender-related patterns have been replicated all around the planet, however, the virulence with influenza struck varied from place to place. Inhabitants of particular parts of Asia have been a shocking 30 times more likely to die from the flu than people in areas of Europe. Generally, Asia and Africa suffered maximum death rates, together with the cheapest found in Europe, North America, and Australia. However, there was great variation in continents, also. African countries south of the Sahara experienced death speeds two or even three times greater than those north of the desert, whereas Spain listed among the maximum passing rates in Europe -- double that in Britain, three times that in Denmark. The unevenness did not stop there. Generally, cities endured worse than rural places, but a few cities endured worse than many others, and there was also variation in towns. Newly arrived immigrants tended to die more frequently than older, better-established groups, for example. In the countryside, one village might be decimated while another, apparently similar in every way, got away with a light dose.

What Kinds Of People Caught The Spanish Flu?

Influenza appeared to attack with an element of randomness and cruelty. Since adults in their prime died in droves, unlucky communities imploded. Kids were orphaned, older parents made to fend for them. Individuals were at a loss to explain this clear lottery, and it left them profoundly disturbed. Trying to clarify the feeling that it inspired in him, a French physician in the town of Lyons wrote that it had been rather unlike the "gut pangs" he'd experienced while serving at the front. This has been "a more deep pressure, the feeling of some indefinable terror which had taken hold of the people of the city." It was only afterward when epidemiologists zeroed in on the amounts that patterns started to emerge, and the initial elements of justification were set forward. A number of the variability may be explained by inequalities of wealth and caste -- and, to the extent, it represented these variables: skin color, poor diet, crowded living conditions, and limited access to healthcare weakened the constitution, which makes the poor, immigrants, and cultural minorities more prone to disease. As French historian Patrick Zylberman said: "The virus may have behaved 'democratically,' but the culture it assaulted was hardly egalitarian."

Any other underlying disorder made someone more vulnerable to the Spanish flu, whereas previous exposure to influenza itself modulates the seriousness of a situation. Remote communities without much historic experience of this illness suffered badly, as did cities that were bypassed by the first wave of the pandemic because they were not immunologically 'primed' to the second. As an instance, Rio de Janeiro – the capital of Brazil at the time – received only one wave of flu in October 1918, and experienced a death rate two or three times higher than that recorded in American cities to the north that had received both the spring and autumn waves. And Bristol Bay in Alaska was spared before early 1919, but if the virus eventually gained a foothold it decreased the bay Eskimo inhabitants by 40 percent. Public health efforts made a difference, in spite of the fact that medics didn't know the reason for the disease. Since time immemorial, if contagion is a danger individuals have practiced 'social distancing' -- knowing unconsciously that steering clear of contaminated people increases the prospect of staying healthy. Back in 1918, social distancing took the kind of quarantine zones, isolation wards, and prohibitions on mass parties; in which they had been correctly enforced, these steps slowed the spread. Australia maintained out the autumn wave completely by implementing a successful quarantine in its ports. Exceptions demonstrated the rule. Back in 1918, Persia was a collapsed country after decades of being used as a pawn in the 'Great Game' -- that the battle between the British and the Russians for control of this huge region between the Arabian and Caspian Seas. Its government was weak and almost broke, and it lacked a coherent sanitary infrastructure. Therefore, whenever the flu faded from the northeastern holy city of Mashhad in August 1918, no social distancing measures were enforced. In a fortnight every house and place of business from Mashhad had been infected, and also two-thirds of this city's inhabitants fell ill that autumn. With no limitations on motion, influenza spread thickly with pilgrims, soldiers, and retailers to the four corners of the nation. From now Persia was free of influenza, it had dropped between 8% and 22 percent of its own population (that doubt representing the fact that, in a state in crisis, collecting statistics was barely a priority). Even 8 percent equates to the mortality rate in Ireland.

Where disparities in rates of illness and death were perceived, people's explanations reflected contemporary understanding – or, rather, misunderstanding – of infectious disease. When Charles Darwin laid out his theory of evolution by natural selection in *On the Origin of Species* (1859), he had not intended his ideas to be applied to human societies, but others of his time did just that, creating the 'science' of eugenics. Eugenicists believed that mankind included 'races' and from 1918 their thinking was mainstream. Some eugenicists noticed that sectors of society suffered against influenza, which they credited to some inferiority. They'd incorporated germ theory in their world perspective: when the poor and the working classes were prone to disease, concluded the eugenicists, they only had themselves to blame, since Pasteur had instructed that disease was preventable.

Indian Anxieties

The consequences of the line of thinking are exemplified in India. That land's British colonizers had long taken the view that India was inherently unhygienic, and so had invested little in indigenous healthcare. As many as 18 million Indians died in the pandemic -- that the reduction in numbers of any nation on the planet. However, there was a backlash. Resentment was fueled by the British reply to the spread of influenza. Tensions came to a head with the passage in 1919. This triggered calm protests, and on 13 April British troops fired into an unarmed crowd in Amritsar, murdering countless Indian individuals -- a massacre that galvanized the liberty movement. Uprisings were prompted by influenza elsewhere. The fall of 1918 saw a tide of workers' strikes and protests around the world. Disgruntlement was smoldering since prior to the Russian revolutions of 1917, but influenza fanned the flames by exacerbating what was a dire source situation, also by highlighting inequality. Even well-ordered Switzerland narrowly prevented a civil war in November 1918 following leftwing groups attributed to a large number of influenza deaths from the military on the authorities and army control. There were regions of the planet where individuals hadn't heard of Darwin or germ theory, and in which the people turned into explanations that are more tried-and-tested. From the rural interior of China, as an instance, a lot of individuals still thought that illness had been sent by dragons and demons; they paraded amounts of dinosaurs through the roads in the hope of appeasing the irate spirits. A missionary physician explained going from house to house in Shanxi province in early 1919, and locating scissors put indoors "to ward off demons or perchance to cut them in 2". In the west that was modernized, individuals vacillated death often seemed to strike without rhyme or reason. Many still remembered a more mystical, pre-Darwinian era, and four years of war had worn down psychological defenses. Seeing how their men of science were to assist them, most people came to think that the stunt was an act of god retribution because of their sins. In Zamora -- exactly the exact same Spanish town whose paper said with such confidence the representative of disorder had been Pfeiffer's bacillus -- that the bishop defied the health authorities' ban on mass parties and ordered people to the dinosaurs to placate "God's legitimate anger." This town then recorded among the maximum death tolls from influenza in Spain -- a simple fact of which its inhabitants were conscious, even though they do not appear to have held it from their own bishop. They gave him a trophy in recognition of his attempts to end his or her suffering. This illustrates gulfs were represented by answers to influenza. The 1918 pandemic struck a planet, which was completely unprepared for this, dealing a body blow to scientific hubris, and destabilizing political and social orders for decades ahead.

Chapter - 5 Kinds Of Influenza Viruses

There are four kinds of influenza viruses: A, B, C, and D. Human influenza A, and B viruses cause seasonal epidemics of illness (called the flu season) nearly every winter in the USA. Influenza A virus is the sole flu virus known to induce flu pandemics, i.e., worldwide epidemics of influenza disease. A pandemic can happen when a new, distinct influenza virus emerges, which both infects individuals and has the capacity to spread efficiently between individuals. Influenza type C cause illness and aren't believed to trigger influenza epidemics. Cattle affect aren't known to infect or cause illness in humans. Flu viruses are divided into subtypes based on two proteins on the surface of the virus: hemagglutinin (H) and neuraminidase (N). There are 18 distinct hemagglutinin subtypes and 11 distinct neuraminidase subtypes (H1 via H18 and N1 via N11, respectively). Just 131 subtypes have been discovered in character when there are 198 influenzas A subtype mixes. Present-day subtypes of flu A viruses which routinely circulate in people contain A (H1N1) and A (H3N2). Influenza A subtypes could be further broken down into distinct genetic "clades" and "sub-clades." Watch the "Influenza Viruses" picture below to get a visual depiction of those classifications.

Human Seasonal Influenza Viruses

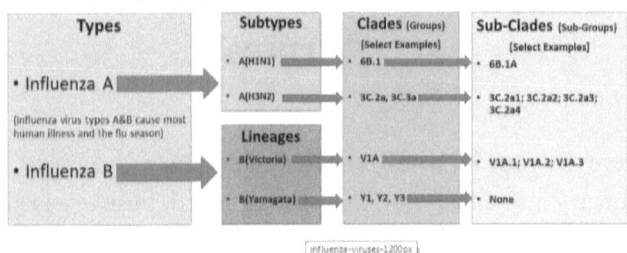

This graphic shows the two types of influenza viruses (A,B) that cause most human illness and that are responsible for the flu season each year. Influenza A viruses are further classified into subtypes, while influenza B viruses are further classified into two lineages: B/Yamagata and B/Victoria. Both influenza A and B viruses can be further classified into specific clades and sub-clades (which are sometimes called groups and sub-groups).

Clades and sub-clades could be rather called "classes" and "sub-groups," respectively. An influenza clade or band is a further subdivision of influenza viruses (past subtypes or lineages) dependent on the similarity of the HA receptor sequences. (Watch the Genome Sequencing and Genetic Characterization page for more info). Clades and subclades are revealed on phylogenetic trees as forms of viruses that normally have comparable genetic changes (i.e., nucleotide or amino acid changes) and also have one common ancestor represented as a node in the tree (see Figure 1). Dividing viruses to clades and subclades enables flu specialists to monitor the ratio of viruses from various clades inflow. Be aware that clades and sub-clades which are genetically distinct from others aren't necessarily antigenically distinct (i.e. viruses out of a particular clade or sub-clade might not have changes that affect host resistance compared with other clades or sub-clades). Currently circulating influenza A(H1N1) viruses are about the pandemic 2009 H1N1 virus, which arose in the spring of 2009 and caused an influenza pandemic (CDC 2009

60

H1N1 Flu site). This virus clinically referred to as the "A (H1N1) pdm09 virus," and more commonly called "2009 H1N1," has continued to float since then. All these H1N1 viruses have experienced relatively small genetic modifications and modifications to their antigenic properties (i.e., the properties of this virus that influence resistance) as time passes. Of all of the flu viruses which habitually circulate and cause illness in people, influenza A (H3N2) viruses have a tendency to change more quickly, both genetically and antigenically. Influenza A (H3N2) viruses have shaped many different, genetically distinct clades lately, which continue to co-circulate. Influenza B viruses aren't divided into subtypes, but rather are categorized into two lineages: B/Yamagata and B/Victoria. Influenza B viruses may be classified into sub-clades and clades. Influenza B viruses normally change more gradually when it comes to their genetic and antigenic properties compared to influenza A viruses, particularly influenza A(H3N2) viruses. Influenza surveillance data in the last years reveals the co-circulation of influenza B viruses from the lineages from the USA and across the world. The proportion of influenza B viruses that circulate may vary by location.

Influenza Vaccine Viruses

One influenza A (H1N1), one influenza A (H3N2), and one or 2 Influenza B viruses (depending upon the vaccine) are contained in every year's flu vaccines. Obtaining a flu vaccine may protect against influenza viruses, which are similar to the viruses used to make disease. Info concerning the vaccine of this season is located at preventing Seasonal Flu with Vaccination. Influenza vaccines don't protect against flu D or C viruses. Additionally, influenza vaccines won't protect against disease and illness due to other viruses, which also may lead to influenza-like symptoms. There are a number of different viruses besides flu that may lead to influenza-like illness (ILI) that disperse during the influenza season.

Influenza Virus Subtypes

The term 'flu' is used for almost any respiratory illness with systemic disorders, which might be caused by a plethora of viral or bacterial agents in addition to influenza viruses. But, true flu is a serious infectious disease brought on by a member of the orthomyxovirus family, including influenza viruses A, B, and C. Influenza outbreaks generally occur in winter in temperate climates. In the USA, the flu season starts in October or November and peaks between March and December. Important outbreaks of flu are connected with influenza virus type A or B. Influenza A infects birds, people, swine, horses, dogs, and seals. Influenza A is accountable for regular, generally annual outbreaks or epidemics of varying seriousness, and intermittent pandemics, whereas influenza B triggers outbreaks each two to four decades. Influenza B viruses create exactly the identical spectrum of disease as influenza A. However, influenza B viruses don't cause pandemics, maybe because they mostly infect people and rarely infect animals. Nearly all adults are infected with the influenza C virus, which induces respiratory tract disease that was moderate. Lower respiratory tract infections are infrequent.

Flu viruses are Classified with the following advice:

• Form A, B or C/place isolated/number of all isolate/year isolated

• Influenza A is split into subtypes based on their hemagglutinin (H) and neuraminidase (N) proteins. There are 16 H and 9 N variations, but every virus has just 1 H and an N variation.

The influenza virus is an enveloped virus, meaning that the outer layer is a lipid membrane which the virus acquires from the host cell. Inserted into the lipid membrane will be the viral glycoprotein, hemagglutinin (H) and neuraminidase (N). Influenza A virions have three membrane proteins (H, N, and M2), whilst Influenza B virions have four (H, N, NB, and BM2). Under the lipid membrane is your M1 viral matrix protein that offers strength and rigidity into the viral envelope. The M2 protein is a proton station that's the goal of these antiviral drugs amantadine and rimantadine. Within influenza, B, or A virion are eight sections of viral RNA that take all of the genetic information required to synthesize new virus contamination. These RNA sections are tagged HA (hemagglutinin), NA (neuraminidase), PB1, PB2, PA, NP, M, and NS. Antigens on the inner proteins M1 and NP are type-specific and utilized to ascertain whether a specific flu virus is type A, B, or C. The two M1 and NP proteins of members of every kind display cross reactivity. Hemagglutinin is a surface glycoprotein that binds to sialic acid residues to epithelial cell surface glycoprotein. This interaction is essential for attachment and fusion of viral and cell membranes that are senile. Neuraminidase digests sialic acid (neuraminic acid) on the surface of cells, boosting entry of the virus to the cell. Neuraminidase facilitates penetration of the mucous coating in the lymph nodes. By late disease, virtually all sialic acid was taken away from infected cell surface, which makes it is simpler to get progeny virions to disseminate to other tissues. N is the goal of these anti-inflammatory drugs Relenza and Tamiflu.

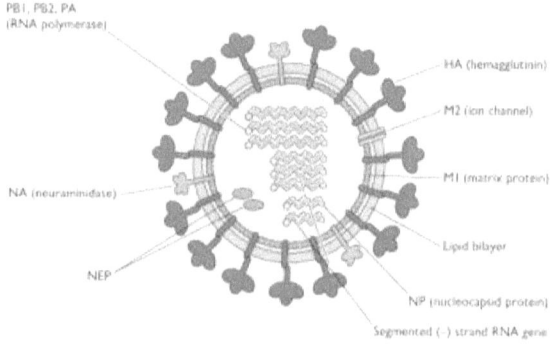

Influenza C viruses tend to be somewhat distinct. They contain 7 RNA segments rather than eight. The significant influenza C virus glycoprotein is known as HEF (hemagglutinin-esterase-fusion) since it has the functions of both the N and H. A small viral envelope protein is CM2, which acts as an ion channel. N and H display more antigenic variation compared to inner proteins and would be the significant determinants of both Influenza A subtype along with strain-specificity. Together with 16 H and 9 N, you will find 144 potential subtypes of influenza A. Minor changes in the envelope glycoprotein, hemagglutinin, and neuraminidase, are known as antigenic drift, and significant changes are known as antigenic shifts.

Antigenic drifts are connected with localized outbreaks, while antigenic changes are correlated with epidemics and pandemics of Influenza A. Antigenic drift is because of a point mutation at HA or NA. Inefficient proofreading by Influenza viral RNA polymerase leads to a high prevalence of transcription mistakes and amino acid substitutions from hemagglutinin or neuraminidase, enabling new versions to prevent preexisting humoral resistance and lead to Influenza outbreaks. An individual resistant to the initial strain isn't resistant to the drifted one. The antigenic shift is because of HA or NA gene reassortment which ends in the synthesis of H or N protein variations. Wild birds are the natural hosts of influenza A virus, for many subtypes. Pigs also play an essential part in the growth of human pandemic strains since pig trachea comprises receptors for both avian and human influenza viruses, and reptiles encourage the development of both kinds of viruses. Genetic reassortment between avian and human virus might occur in cows, resulting in a novel strain. When a pig gets infected with both human and avian viruses, then the RNAs of both viruses have been duplicated in the nucleus. When new virus particles are constructed in the cell membrane, a number of these RNA segments can arise from both of the infecting viruses. New viruses that inherit RNA from the avian and human flu are known as reassortants. They may comprise creature and human proteins H or N. Whether this virus reassortant can infect people, they are going to have little resistance to it, raising the odds of an outbreak or pandemic. The H1N1 pandemic, which happened in 2009, was because of the reassortment of avian, human, and swine influenza viruses.

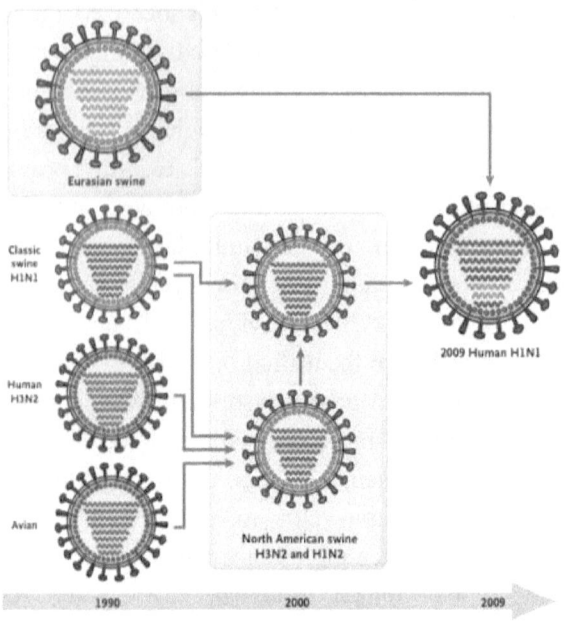

Reassortment can happen between influenza viruses of this same kind. Why influenza A viruses never swap RNA sections with influenza B or B 18 isn't known. Influenza B is not as prone to undergo antigenic change because there's not an animal reservoir for this virus.

Human Influenza

Even though nine N virus subtypes and 16 H happen in their Natural reservoir of aquatic creatures, just three hemagglutinin subtypes (H1, H2, and H3) and two neuraminidase subtypes (N1 and N2) have demonstrated stable lineages in people and generated widespread human respiratory disease. Today H3N2 and h1N1 cause epidemics. Changes have been responsible. The extremely severe outbreak of 1918 and 1919 (swine flu or Spanish flu) has been connected with the development of antigenic changes in both hemagglutinin (H1) and neuraminidase (N1) of influenza A. Between 50 and 100 million people were killed by this virus. The H1N1 virus responsible was derived from an avian strain that adapted to infect and efficiently transmit between humans. A lot of flu pandemics have occurred throughout the 20th century in people. In 1957, a change was made by a reassortant. This virus has been known as influenza since it originated in China and then spread worldwide. It caused between 4 and 1 million deaths and continued until 1958. Back in 1968, another human-avian reassortant generated an antigenic change from H2N2 into H3N2 (Hong Kong flu). Considering that the change involved hemagglutinin, this outbreak was less extensive, inducing 750,000 deaths. H3N2 influenza A reoccurred in 2006 and late 2003. It's now endemic in both pig and individual populations. The resistance to the virus has risen from 1 percent in 1994.

In 1977, an influenza A was generated by people who lacked preexisting resistance were influenced by that to H1N1. Since the late 1990s, reassortant swine influenza, A virus genes from swine, human, and avian strains of influenza, have been detected among swine herds in North America. Back in an epidemic of H1N1, March 2009 Influenza A virus has been discovered in Mexico that propagates States, Canada, and the world. The pandemic was announced to be over in August 2010. A reassortment of 2 caused this pandemic. Strains that are swine, one anxiety that is human, and yet another avian strain of influenza. The virus was known as Swine Flu since the proportion of genes originated from swine Influenza viruses. In reaction to this possibility of a pandemic, a vaccination campaign employing a monovalent vaccine has been undertaken. Even though The WHO announced that this pandemic over this H1N1 strain proceeds to circulate around the world together with influenza. H1N1 was comprised of the influenza vaccine that is 2011. Influenza A viruses, which people may be infected by circulating in creatures. These germs are known to as "version influenza viruses" and, as an abbreviation, will be designated using a "v." As of December 23, 2011, the Centers for Disease Control and Prevention (CDC) has received reports of 35 instances of human disease with esophageal origin variant flu viruses since 2005. The frequency with which these variant influenza viruses have been detected has increased since 2011. In the past 6 months of 2011, 12 US inhabitants in five distinct countries (Indiana, Iowa, Maine, Pennsylvania, and West Virginia) have been discovered to be infected with this specific influenza A version virus, which had genes in human flu, swine, and avian viruses. This virus differs from the other cases because it has acquired another genetic change, the matrix (M) gene from the 2009 H1N1 pandemic virus. Currently, nobody knows what the M gene's accession means in relation to disease severity or transmissibility in humans. So far, sickness associated with this particular virus has been self-limited and light. Restricted serologic studies conducted at CDC imply that adults might have some preexisting resistance to H3N2v kids don't. The next diagram demonstrates how the virus generated from the reassortment of this matrix. (M) Gene segments in the 2009 H1N1 virus that is pandemic using

the HA and NA gene Segments in the Swine H3N2
reassortment virus in 1998 -- 2011.

Construction And Genetics

Influenza type A viruses are extremely similar in
construction to Influenza viruses forms B, C, and D. The
virus particle (also referred to as the virion) is 80-120
nanometers in diameter like the tiniest virions embrace an
elliptical form. Every particle's duration may be in excess
of thousands of micrometers, making virions, and
fluctuates because of the fact that flu is Pleomorphic.
Confusion regarding the nature of the Influenza virus
pleomorphic originates from the observation that
laboratory-adapted strains normally decrease the ability to
make filaments and these laboratory-adapted strains were
the first to be visualized by electron microscopy. Despite
these shapes, viruses are similar in makeup. They're all
composed of an envelope comprising two kinds of
proteins. Both big proteins found in the exterior of viral
contaminants are hemagglutinin (HA) and neuraminidase
(NA). HA is a protein that mediates the binding of the
virion to the target entrance and cells of the viral genome.
NA is included in discharge in the abundant attachment
websites within mucus in addition to the release of virions
from cells that were infected. These proteins are the targets
for drugs. Furthermore, they are also the antigen proteins
to which a host's antibodies can bind and trigger an
immune response. Influenza type A viruses have been
categorized into subtypes based on the face of the
envelope. You will find 9 subtypes of NA understood and
16 subtypes of HA, but H 1, 3, and 2, and N 2 and 1 are

found in people. The core of a virion includes other proteins that protect and pack the material and the genome. Unlike the genomes of most organisms (such as humans, plants, animals, and bacteria) that are composed of double-stranded DNA, several viral genomes comprise another, single-stranded nucleic acid known as RNA. Unusually for a virus the influenza type A virus genome isn't a single bit of RNA, but rather, it is composed of segmented parts of negative-sense RNA: every piece comprising either a couple of genes that code for a gene product (protein). The expression negative-sense RNA just suggests the RNA genome cannot be translated into protein straight; it should first be transcribed to positive-sense RNA before it can be translated into protein solutions. The nature of the genome allows for the exchange of genes between different strains.

The entire Influenza A virus genome is 13,588 bases long and is contained on eight RNA segments that code for at least 10 but up to 14 proteins, depending on the strain. The significance of the existence of alternative gene products may differ:

• Segment 1 encodes RNA polymerase subunit (PB2).

• Segment 2 Fragrant RNA polymerase subunit (PB1) and also the PB1-F2 protein, which induces cell death, using different reading frames from precisely the exact same RNA segment.

• Segment 3 encodes RNA polymerase subunit (PA) and the PA-X protein, which has a role in host transcription shutoff.

• Segment 4 encodes for HA (hemagglutinin). Approximately 500 molecules of hemagglutinin are essential to creating 1 virion. HA determines the seriousness and the scope of a viral disease in a host organism.

• Segment 5 encodes NP, which is a nucleoprotein.

• Segment 6 encodes NA (neuraminidase). Approximately 100 molecules of neuraminidase are essential to creating 1 virion.

• Segment 7 encodes two matrix proteins (M1 and M2) using different reading frames from precisely the exact same RNA segment. About 3,000 matrix protein molecules are essential to creating 1 virion.

• Segment 8 encodes two different non-structural proteins (NS1 and NEP) using different reading frames from precisely the exact same RNA segment.

The RNA segments of the genome have foundation sequences in the terminal endings, letting them bond. Transcription of the viral (-) sense genome (v RNA) can only move following the PB2 protein binds to host restricted RNAs, allowing for the PA subunit to cleave several nucleotides following the cap. This cap and nucleotides that are accompanied function as the primer for transcription initiation. Transcription proceeds across the vRNA before a stretch of many Uralic bases is attained, initiating a 'stuttering' where the viral mRNA is poly-adenylated, making a mature transcript for nuclear export and translation by sponsor machines. While the synthesis of proteins occurs in the cytoplasm, the RNA synthesis occurs from the cell nucleus. When the viral proteins have been built into virions, the constructed virions leave the nucleus and migrate to the cell membrane. [32] The host cell membrane contains stains of viral transmembrane proteins (HA, NA, and M2) and an underlying layer of the M1 protein that helps the constructed virions to bud throughout the membrane, releasing completed enveloped viruses to the extracellular fluid.

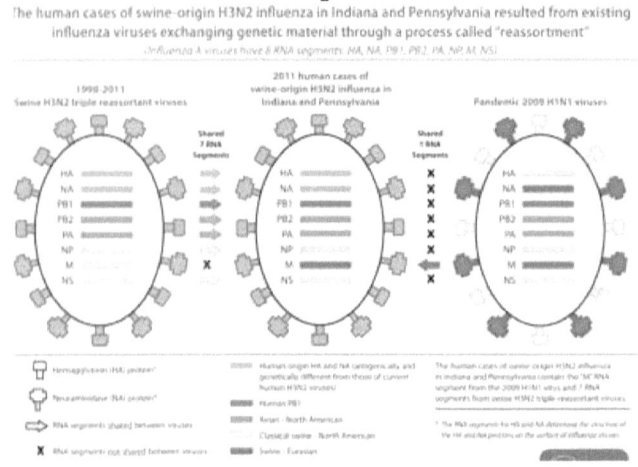

The human cases of swine-origin H3N2 influenza in Indiana and Pennsylvania resulted from existing influenza viruses exchanging genetic material through a process called "reassortment"

Influenza A (H3N2) v viruses discovered thus far are vulnerable Into oseltamivir (Tamiflu®) or zanamivir (Relenza®). As these viruses possess the gene in the influenza A (H1N1) pdm09 virus, they are resistant to amantadine and rimantadine.

Avian Influenza

Viruses that infect domestic or wild birds Cause limited illness. But, properties that have made them more virulent have been obtained by viruses inside the H5 and H7 subtypes. Avian H5N1 influenza A viruses have been endemic among poultry and bird populations, and therefore are regarded as the world's leading flu pandemic threat. The primary institution of avian influenza H5N1 with clinical respiratory disease happened in Hong Kong in 1997 through a poultry epidemic of highly pathogenic H5N1 flu in live-bird markets. This epidemic was associated with a mortality rate and a high prevalence of pneumonia. All virus genes were indicating that the species barrier had jumped. Surveillance showed evidence of transmission, and no cases were reported after the culling of poultry. Since its development in humans in 1997, influenza H5N1 has experienced antigenic drift. H5N1 virus seems to have expanded its host array besides infecting humans and poultry. Fatal disease in cats was reported. There are no reports of cats distributing the virus. All human H5 infections have caused viruses to own the subtype. Concern remains that this strain may mutate, or experience reassortment and get the ability to spread from human to human. Avian influenza H7 viruses also have been associated with the disorder that was occasional. Subtype H7 viruses with numerous N subtypes (N2, N3, and N7) have transmitted from birds to people. Outbreaks of H7N7 occurred among poultry in the Netherlands. Employees had grown influenza-like disease and conjunctivitis. Infections are reported among poultry workers in Italy, the USA, Canada, and the United Kingdom. Much like H5N1, all genes in the viruses have been avian in origin. Avian H9N2 viruses are endemic in poultry in Asia and are isolated from cows. By kids with moderate respiratory disease, influenza H9N2 viruses have been isolated back in Hong Kong in 1999, 2003, 2007, and 2009. The viruses are responsible for the 1999 ailments comprised enzymes homologous, implying that these strains roseby reassortment.

Kinds Of Flu

Not all influenza areequal. Some forms can make you quite sick, though milder symptoms are caused by other kinds of influenza. Keep reading to learn about different kinds of flu.

How Can A Flu Virus Make Me Sick?

Flu viruses enter the body through your nose, mouth, or eyes. Every time you touch your hands you're possibly infecting yourself. This makes it important to keep your palms virus-free with thorough and regular hand washing. Advise relatives to do the exact same to protect against the flu.

What Are The Different Types Of Flu?

There are 3 Kinds of influenza viruses: A, B, and C. Type A And B trigger the yearly flu epidemics, which have around 20 percent of the populace sniffling, coughing, and conducting high fevers. Form C also causes influenza. Type C influenza symptoms are not as severe. The flu is related to 49,000 deaths and between 3,000 and 200,000 hospitalizations every year. The influenza vaccine was produced to attempt and prevent these epidemics.

What's Type A Flu?

Type influenza or flu Animals, even though it is common for individuals to endure the ailments related to this kind of flu. Wild birds act as hosts because of this particular flu virus. Type A influenza virus is continually changing and is normally responsible for the huge flu epidemics. The influenza A2 virus (along with other forms of flu) is spread by those that are infected. The most common flu hot spots are those surfaces that an infected person has touched and rooms where he or she has been recently, especially areas where he or she has been sneezing.

What's Type B Flu? Type B influenza is located in
humans. Type B influenza might cause a less intense response than type A influenza virus, but sometimes type B influenza may still be extremely dangerous. Influenza type B viruses aren't categorized by subtype and don't cause pandemics.

How Is Type C Flu Virus Different From Others?

Influenza C viruses are found in humans. They're milder than type A or B. People do not become very ill in the flu type C viruses. Type C influenza viruses cause epidemics that do not cause epidemics.

Do Different Kinds Of Flu Viruses Reach The Population Every Year?

Various strains of influenza replace the strains of this

virus. That is the reason it's important to have a flu shot every year to make sure your entire body develops resistance to the latest strains of this virus. According to the CDC, the viruses at a flu shot and Flu Mist vaccine may change annually based on international surveillance and scientists' estimations about which types and strains of influenza will probably be potent annually. Formerly, all influenza vaccines protected against three flu viruses: 1 Influenza A (H3N2) virus, 1 Influenza A (H1N1) virus, and one Influenza B virus. Now, Flu Mist, plus a few conventional flu shots, normally cover around four strains: 2 Influenza A viruses along with 2 Influenza B viruses. Approximately two weeks after having a flu shot or Flu Mist, antibodies that provide protection from the influenza viruses grow inside the human body. Nevertheless, Flu Mist is also not suggested for use throughout the 2017-2018 season since it may not be powerful.

What's The Bird Flu?

Bird flu is caused by the influenza virus. Birds can be infected by all its subtypes and influenza A viruses. Birds aren't capable of carrying type C or B flu viruses. There are three subtypes of avian influenza. Even the subtypes H5 and H7 are the most deadly, although the H9 subtype is not as dangerous.

Which Kind Of Bird Flu Is In The News?

Health care professionals were quite vocal regarding the strain of avian influenza called H5N1. The main reason H5N1 has caused so much alarm is the way it can maneuver from wild birds to poultry, then on to individuals. While wild birds are generally resistant to the catastrophic and potentially deadly consequences of H5N1, the virus has killed over half of those people infected with it. The possibility of avian flu is usually low in the majority of people since the virus doesn't normally infect humans. Infections have occurred as the result of contact with infected birds. The spread of the disease from humans to humans has been reported to be quite rare.

Should I Understand Catching Bird Flu?

Individuals in the USA have less to fear than individuals who live overseas. The majority of the illnesses have been reported among those who've had contact with farm animals in nations. Additionally, individuals aren't able to capture the bird influenza virus from eating cooked chicken, turkey, or duck. The virus is killed by high temperatures.

Is There A Vaccine For Bird Flu?

No. It's crucial that you know the influenza vaccine doesn't offer protection against bird flu or avian flu.

Influenza Type A Viruses

There are four kinds of influenza viruses: A, B, C, and D. Wild aquatic birds -- especially specific wild ducks, geese, swans, gulls, shorebirds and terns -- would be the natural hosts for many flu types A viruses.

Subtypes Of Influenza A Infection

Influenza A viruses are divided into subtypes on the basis of two proteins on the surface of the virus: hemagglutinin (HA) and neuraminidase (NA). There are 11 NA subtypes and 18 known HA subtypes. Many distinct combinations of HA and NA proteins are possible. For example, an "H7N2 virus" designates the influenza A virus subtype that has an HA 7 protein and an NA two protein. In the same way, an "H5N1" virus has an HA 5 protein and an NA 1 protein. All known subtypes of influenza A viruses can infect birds, except subtypes H17N10 and H18N11; that has just been discovered in rodents. Just two influenza A virus subtypes (i.e., H1N1, and H3N2) are now in general circulation among individuals. Some subtypes are located in animal species that were contaminated. Some subtypes are found in other infected animal species. For example, H7N7 and H3N8 virus infections can cause illness in horses, and H3N8 virus infection causes illness in horses and dogs.

Lineages Of Influenza A Infection

Avian influenza (AI) viruses – influenza viruses that infect birds – have evolved into distinct genetic lineages in different geographic locations. These various lineages may be distinguished by analyzing the hereditary make-up of those viruses. By way of instance, AI viruses circulating in birds from Asia, known as Oriental lineage AI viruses, could be considered genetically distinct from AI viruses that circulate among birds in North America (known as North American lineage AI viruses). These wide lineage classifications could be further narrowed by genetic comparisons that enable researchers to set the many closely-related viruses collectively. Therefore, the North American lineage of all H7N9 viruses might be further broken down to the North American 'wild bird' lineage versus the North American 'poultry' lineage. The hosts, time period, and geographic location are frequently utilized in the lineage title to assist further delineate 1 lineage from the other.

Highly Pathogenic And Low Pathogenic Avian Influenza A Viruses

Avian flu A viruses have been designated as highly pathogenic avian influenza (HPAI) or very low pathogenicity avian influenza (LPAI) based on molecular features of the virus and the capability of the virus to cause illness and mortality in cows at a lab setting. HPAI and LPAI designations don't refer to the seriousness of the disease in cases of human infection with these viruses; both LPAI and HPAI viruses have caused acute illness in humans. Poultry infected with LPAI viruses might show no symptoms of a disorder or just exhibit mild illness (such as ruffled feathers and a drop in egg production) that might not be discovered. The infection of poultry together with HPAI viruses can result in severe illness. The two LPAI and HPAI viruses could propagate quickly through poultry flocks. HPAI virus disease can lead to disease that affects multiple internal organs together with mortality around 90% to 100% in cows, often within two days. Ducks may be infected with no symptoms of illness. There are genetic and antigenic differences between the flu A virus subtypes that normally infect creatures and the ones that could infect birds and humans. Avian flu viruses infect individuals. The most often identified subtypes of avian flu that have caused human infections are H5, H7, and H9 viruses. Other viruses, such as H10N8, H10N7, and H6N8, are discovered in humans but to a lesser degree.

Influenza A H5

There are known subtypes of H5 (H5N1, H5N2, H5N3, H5N4, H5N5, H5N6, H5N7, H5N8, and H5N9). Many H5 viruses found globally in wild fish and birds are LPAI, but sometimes HPAI viruses are detected. A sporadic H5 virus disease of people has happened, for example, with Asian lineage because HPAI H5N1 viruses are now circulating among poultry in Asia and the Middle East. Human infection of H5N1 virus infections is reported in 16 states, often leading to acute pneumonia and higher than 50% mortality.

Influenza A H7

There are known subtypes of (H7N1, H7N2, H7N3, H7N4, H7N5, H7N6, H7N7, H7N8, and H7N9). H7 viruses found in wild fish and birds are LPAI viruses.

Virus disease in humans is rare. The most often identified H7 viruses associated with human disease are lineage avian influenza A (H7N9) viruses, which have been detected in China in 2013. While human infections are infrequent, these have resulted in acute respiratory illness and passing. Along with Asian H7N9 viruses, H7N7 virus diseases are reported. These viruses have mostly induced mild to moderate illness in humans, with symptoms that have conjunctivitis or upper respiratory tract ailments.

Influenza A H9

There are known subtypes of H9 (H9N1, H9N2, H9N3, H9N4, H9N5, H9N6, H9N7, H9N8, and H9N9); all of the H9 viruses identified globally in wild fish and birds are LPAI viruses. The virus has been found in bird populations in Africa, Europe, the Middle East, and Asia. Unusual, intermittent H9N2 virus infections in people are reported to normally cause mild upper respiratory tract disease; one disease has led to death.

Chapter - 6 The Flu Season

While seasonal influenza (flu) viruses have been detected year-round in the USA, influenza viruses are most frequent during winter and the autumn. Flu activity starts to rise in October, although the time and duration of influenza seasons may vary. Most of the time flu activity peaks between December and February, although activity can last as late as May. The figure below reveals flu action in the United States. The "peak month of flu activity" is the month with the highest percentage of respiratory specimens testing positive for influenza virus infection during that influenza season. During this 36-year period, flu activity most often peaked in February (15 seasons), followed by December (7 seasons), January (6 seasons), and March (6 seasons).

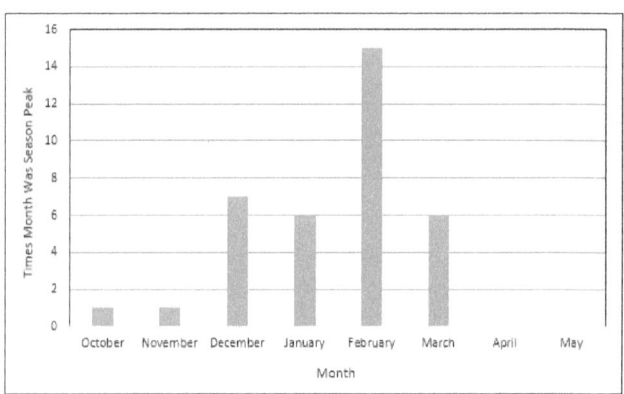

When Is The Flu Season In The USA?

In the USA, flu season happens in the autumn and winter. While flu viruses circulate year-round, the majority of the time influenza action peaks between February and December, however, action can last as late as May. The general health impact (e.g., infections, hospitalizations, and deaths) of a flu season fluctuates from season to season. CDC collects, compiles, and analyzes information on flu action year-long in the USA and generates Flu View, a weekly surveillance report, and Flu View Interactive, allowing for much more in-depth exploration of flu surveillance information. The Weekly U.S. Influenza Summary Update is updated each week from October through May.

How Can CDC Track The Development Of The Influenza Season?

The general health impact (e.g., infections, hospitalizations, and deaths) of a flu season fluctuates from season to season. CDC collects, compiles, and analyzes data on a surveillance report flu action yearlong in the USA and produces FluView, a weekly surveillance report, and FluView Interactive, which allows for a more in-depth exploration of influenza surveillance data. The Weekly U.S. Influenza Summary Update is updated every week from October through May. The U.S. flu surveillance process is a collaborative effort between CDC and its numerous partners in local and state health departments, public health and medical labs, vital statistics offices, healthcare providers, and practices and emergency departments. Info in five classes is gathered from eight Distinct data sources which enable CDC to:

•   Learn where and when influenza activity is happening

•   Track influenza-related disease

•   Determine what flu viruses have been circulating

•   Detect changes in flu viruses

•   Assess the impact the flu is having to hospitalizations and deaths from the USA

These surveillance elements allow CDC to determine if and where influenza activity is currently happening, determine what kinds of flu viruses are currently circulating, detect changes in the flu viruses examined and collected, assess the effect of flu, and monitor patterns of disease. All influenza activity reporting by states, laboratories, and health care providers is voluntary. For more information about CDC's influenza surveillance activities, see the Overview of Influenza Surveillance in the United States.

Why Can There Be A Week-Long Lag Between The Information And As Soon As It's Documented?

Influenza surveillance information collection relies on a reporting. It starts on Sunday and ends on the Saturday of every week. Each surveillance player is asked to outline the information that was weekly and submit an application to the CDC. The data is downloaded, compiled, and analyzed in the CDC. The data is utilized to upgrade Flu View Interactive and FluView.

Do Other Respiratory Viruses Circulate Throughout The Influenza Season?

In addition to flu viruses, several other respiratory viruses also circulate during the flu season and can cause symptoms and illnesses similar to those seen with flu infection. These respiratory viruses comprise rhinovirus (one reason for this "common cold") and respiratory syncytial virus (RSV), that's the usual cause of acute respiratory disease in young children, in addition to a chief cause of death from respiratory disease in people aged 65 years and older.

When Exactly Is Flu Season?

Although flu season is usually thought of as occurring in the winter, the severity and timing vary from year to year. To best protect you no matter the particular interval, the Centers for Disease Control and Prevention (CDC) recommends getting vaccinated at the end of October.

In general, flu season in the United States can start anytime in late fall, peak in mid-to-late winter (between December and February), and continue through early spring. Flu season lasts about 13 weeks. In a few years it could linger into May, although it is going to finish by April. It's a great idea you receivev the flu shot, but a late influenza shot offers protection when flu season descends into April or even May.

Check Out Past Flu Seasons

The strain of flu that circulates can change from year to year, and the vaccine is adjusted in an attempt to predict which will predominate. Here's a look at the flu within the last 10 years:

2018-2019 Flu Seasons:

• Peak: Mid-February

• Most Frequent strain: Influenza A--both H3N2 and H1N1

2017-2018 Flu Seasons:

• Peak: January and February

• Most Frequent strain: Influenza A (H3N2)

2016-2017 Flu Seasons:

• Peak: Mid-March

• Most Frequent strain: Influenza A (H3N2)

2015-2016 Flu Seasons:

• Peak: Mid-March

• Most Frequent strain: 2009 H1N1 Influenza A

2014-2015 Flu Seasons:

• Peak: overdue December

• Most Frequent strain: Influenza A (H3N2)

2013-2014 Flu Seasons:

- Peak: overdue December

- Most Frequent strain: 2009 H1N1 Influenza A

2012-2013 Flu Seasons:

- Peak: overdue December

- Most Frequent strain: Influenza A (H3N2)

2011-2012 Flu Seasons:

- Peak: Mid-March

- Most Frequent strain: Influenza A (H3N2)

2010-2011 Flu Seasons:

- Peak: Historical February

- Most Frequent strain: Influenza A (H3N2)

Cause

Three virus families, Influenza virus A, B, and C, are the main infective agents that cause influenza. During periods of temperatures, flu cases grow. Despite the higher incidence of manifestations of the flu during the season, the viruses are actually transmitted throughout populations all year round. Every yearly flu season is generally connected with a significant influenza virus subtype. The related subtype affects every year because of the growth of immunological resistance to some preceding year's strain (through vaccinations and vulnerability), and mutational changes in formerly dormant viruses strains.

The Precise mechanism Supporting the character of flu outbreaks is unknown. Some suggested explanations are:

• Individuals are indoors more often during the winter, they are in close contact more often, and this promotes transmission from person to person.

• A seasonal decrease in the quantity of ultraviolet radiation can lessen the probability of the virus being ruined or damaged by direct radiation harm or indirect consequences (i.e. ozone concentration), increasing the probability of infection.

• Cold temperatures contribute to the drier atmosphere, which may dehydrate mucous membranes, preventing the body from effectively defending against respiratory virus infections.

• Viruses are maintained in colder temperatures

because of slower decomposition, allowing them to linger longer on exposed surfaces (doorknobs, countertops, etc.).

•   In countries where children do not go to school in the summer, there is a more pronounced beginning to flu season, coinciding with the start of public school. [citation needed] It is thought that the daycare environment is perfect for the spread of illness.

•   Vitamin D production by Ultraviolet-B from skin impacts the immune system also varies with the seasons.

Research in guinea pigs has shown that the aerosol transmission of the virus is enhanced when the air is cold and dry. The dependence on aridity seems to be a result of degradation of the virus contamination in the atmosphere, while the dependence on chilly appears to be attributed to hosts losing the virus. The investigators didn't find the chilly impaired the guinea pigs' reaction. Research performed by the National Institute of Child Health and Human Development (NICHD) in 2008 discovered that the flu virus has a "butter-like Coating." As it passes the lymph nodes, the coat melts. From the coat becomes a shell. In winter, it can survive in the cold weather very similar to a spore. In the summer, the coating melts before the virus reaches the respiratory tract.

Flu Vaccinations

Flu vaccinations have been used to reduce the effects of the influenza season. Pneumonia vaccinations diminish complications and the ramifications of the influenza season. Since the Northern and Southern Hemisphere has wintered at different times of the year, there are actually two flu seasons each year. Hence, the World Health Organization (aided by the National Influenza Centers) makes two vaccine formulations every year; just one to the Northern, and one to the Southern Hemisphere.

According to the U.S. Department of Health, a growing amount of large businesses provide their workers with seasonal influenza shots, either with a little cost to the worker or as a totally free service. The yearly updated trivalent flu vaccine includes hemagglutinin (HA) surface glycoprotein elements from influenza H3N2, H1N1, and B flu viruses. The strain in January 2006 has been H3N2. Measured resistance to the standard antiviral drugs amantadine and rimantadine in H3N2 has increased from 1% in 1994 to 12% in 2003 to 91% in 2005.

Associated Health Issues

Medical conditions that compromise the immune system increase the risks of flu.

Diabetes

Huge numbers of individuals have diabetes. When blood sugars aren't controlled, diabetics may create a broad variety of complications. Diabetes contributes to elevated blood sugars within the human body, and also this environment permits bacteria and viruses to flourish. If blood sugars have been poorly controlled, moderate flu can easily turn acute, resulting in illness and even death. Uncontrolled blood sugars suppress the immune systems and generally lead to more severe cases of the common cold or influenza. It has been advocated that diabetics have been vaccinated against influenza before the start of the flu season.

Asthma/COPD

It's suggested that asthmatics and COPD patients be vaccinated before the influenza season against influenza. People with asthma may create complications from common cold viruses and flu. Some of the complications include acute respiratory distress syndrome, severe bronchitis, and pneumonia. Every year influenza-related complications in the United States and countless more are observed in the emergency room because of shortness of breath. It's encouraged that asthmatics be vaccinated before the summit of the influenza season, between October and November. Flu vaccine requires about two weeks; it works by boosting the body's immune system.

Cancer

Individuals with cancer have a suppressed immune system. Additionally, many cancer patients undergo radiation treatment and powerful immunosuppressive drugs, which additionally inhibits the body's ability to fight infections. Everybody with cancer can be at risk for complications from influenza and is vulnerable. People with cancer or a history of cancer should receive the seasonal flu shot. As cancer results in complications of hepatitis and pneumonia, the flu vaccination is rigorous for lung cancer sufferers. People with cancer shouldn't get the nasal spray medication. The flu shot is made up of inactivated (killed) viruses, and the nasal spray vaccines are made up of live viruses. The flu shot is much more powerful for people who have a diminished immune system. People who have received cancer treatment, like radiation or chemotherapy treatment over the previous month, or have a blood or lymphatic kind of cancer, must call their physician immediately if they suspect they might have flu.

Hiv/Aids

(HIV) are extremely prone to many different infections. HIV has a huge capability to destroy the human body's immune system and this makes one more prone to not only viral diseases but also fungal, bacterial, and protozoa ailments. People with HIV are at a heightened risk of severe complications. Reports have shown that people with HIV can create cases of pneumonia that require antibiotic treatment and hospitalization. People are at a higher risk of passing and with HIV have an influenza season that is lengthier. Vaccination using the flu shot was proven to increase the immune system and guard against seasonal influenza in certain patients with HIV; people who have HIV should just get vaccinated with the inactivated flu vaccine. Any HIV patient who has been exposed to other people with influenza should see a physician to determine if there is a need for anti-viral medications.

Price

The expense of a flu season in lives lost, medical expenses, and economic impact can be severe.

• "In the USA of America, for instance, recent estimates place the price of flu epidemics into the market at $71-167 billion US dollars annually."

A study estimated that in the United States, annual influenza epidemics result in approximately 600,000 life-years lost, 3 million hospitalized days, and 30 million outpatient visits, resulting in medical costs of $10 billion annually. According to the research, lost earnings due to sickness and loss of life amounted to over $15 billion annually and the overall financial burden of annual flu epidemics figures to over $80 billion. In addition, in the US, the influenza season generally accounts for 200,000 hospitalizations and 41,000 deaths. Since the mortality rate of this H1N1 "swine flu" is significantly lower compared to influenza strains, this amount was reduced in 2009. Based on an article in Clinical Infectious Diseases, printed in 2011, the estimated health burden of 2009 Pandemic Influenza A (H1N1), between April 2009 to April 2010, has been "roughly 60.8 million cases (array: 43.3--89.3 million), 274,304 hospitalizations (195,086--402,719), along with 12,469 deaths (8,868--18,306)" at the USA because of pH1N1."

How Flu Spreads

Person To Person

It can be spread by Individuals with influenza to other people around approximately 6 ft away. Experts believe influenza viruses spread by droplets created when individuals speak, cough, or sneeze. These droplets can land in the mouths or noses of people who are nearby or possibly be inhaled into the lungs. Less often, a person might get the flu by touching a surface or object that has the flu virus on it and then touching their own mouth, nose, or possibly their eyes.

When Flu Spread

Individuals with influenza are contagious in the first three to four days after their illness starts. Most healthy adults may have the ability to infect others beginning 1 day before symptoms develop and up to 5 to 7 days after getting ill. A few individuals with weakened immune systems and kids can pass the virus. Symptoms may start about two times (but may vary from 1 to 4 times) after the virus enters your system. That usually means you might have the ability to pass on the flu to someone else before you know you're sick or while sick. Some people can be infected with the flu virus but have no signs. Those individuals may spread the virus.

Stage Of Contagiousness

You may have the ability to pass the flu to someone else before you understand you're sick.

•   Individuals with influenza are contagious in the first 3-4 days after their illness starts

•   Some otherwise healthy adults may have the ability to infect others beginning 1 day before symptoms develop and up to 5 to 7 days after getting ill

•   Some individuals, particularly young children and individuals with weakened immune systems, may have the ability to infect other people with influenza viruses for an even longer time

Chapter - 7 Spanish Influenza (1918-20): The International Effect Of The Most Significant Flu Pandemic In History

In the past 150 years, the entire world has witnessed unprecedented improvement in wellbeing. The research indicates that in most countries life expectancy, which affects the average age of death, doubled from approximately 40 decades or less to over 80 decades. This wasn't only an accomplishment across these states. Life expectancy has doubled in most areas of the planet. What also stands out is how abrupt and damning negative health events can be. Most striking is that the large, sudden decrease of life expectancy in 1918 brought on by a remarkably deadly flu pandemic known as the famous 'Spanish flu.' To make sense of the fact that life expectancy declined so abruptly, one has to understand what it measures. Term life expectancy, that is the exact title for this step, just examines the mortality pattern in one specific year then catches this picture of public wellbeing as the average age of death using a hypothetical cohort of individuals so that year's mortality routine could stay constant throughout their whole lifetimes. Period life expectancy is a measure of their people's health in 1 year. This flu outbreak was not limited to Spain and it did not even arise there (a recent study from Olson et al. (2005) indicates that the outbreak originated from New York because of signs of a pre-pandemic tide of this virus in that town). Nevertheless, it was called such because Spain was neutral in the First World War (1914-18), which meant it had been free to report the intensity of the outbreak, while nations which were fighting strove to curb reports how the flu affected their inhabitants to keep morale, not seem diminished in the opinion of the enemies. The flu outbreak began in the spring of 1918 from the Northern Hemisphere. The virus spread rapidly and eventually reached all parts of the world: the epidemic became a pandemic. In a much less-connected universe the virus finally reached extremely distant places like the Alaskan wilderness and Samoa at the center of the Pacific islands. While peak mortality was reached in 1918 the pandemic did not end until two years later in late 1920.

The International Death Count Of This Influenza Now

To have a circumstance for the severity of flu pandemics, it might be very helpful to be aware of the departure count of a normal flu season. Estimates for the number of deaths from the flu are approximately 400,000 deaths each year. Paget et al (2019) indicate a mean of 389,000 and having an uncertainty range 294,000 from 518,000.4 This implies that in the past few years, the flu has been responsible for the passing of 0.0052 percent of the world population -- just one individual for every 18,750.5 Even compared with the minimal quote because of the death count of Spanish influenza (17.4 million) this outbreak, over a century past, led to a death rate which has been 182 times greater than the current baseline. Further below I will briefly discuss similarities and differences with the Coronavirus (COVID-19) in 2019/20.

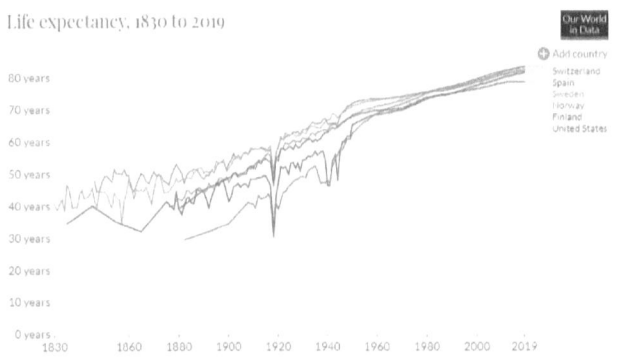

How Many People Died In The Spanish Flu And Other Influenza Pandemics?

Global Deaths Of The Spanish Influenza

Several research groups have worked on the issue that was challenging: reconstructing the health impact of this outbreak. There is now a lot of variability in these estimates and while the academic discussions continue, the range of estimates gives us an understanding of the severity of the event. The visualization here reveals the quotes that are available from the research book. Patterson and Pyle (1991) estimated that between 24.7 and 39.3 million died from the pandemic. The widely cited research by Johnson and Mueller (2002) arrives in a greater estimate of 50 million worldwide deaths. However, the authors suggest that this might be an underestimation and the real death toll was as large as 100 million. The recent analysis by Spreeuwenberg et al. (2018) reasoned that earlier estimates are too large. Their very own quote is 17.4 million deaths.

Global Death Rate

How do these estimates compare with the world's dimensions Population at the moment? How large was the share who died in the pandemic? Estimates imply that the world population in 1918 was 1.8 billion. According to this, the minimal estimate of 17.4 million deaths by Spreeuwenberg et al. (2018) suggests that Spanish influenza killed almost 1 percent (0.95percent) of the world population. If we rely upon the estimate of 50 million deaths released by Johnson and Mueller, it suggests that Spanish influenza killed 2.7 percent of the world population. And when it was actually high -- 100 million since those writers indicate -- then the worldwide death rate could have been 5.4percent. The entire population was rising by approximately 13 million annually in this interval, which suggests the length of the Spanish influenza was probably the last time ever once the world population was declining.

Other Big Flu Pandemics

The Spanish flu pandemic was the largest, but not the only large recent influenza pandemic. Two years before Spanish influenza the Russian influenza pandemic (1889-1894) is thought to have killed 1 million people. Estimates for its death toll of this "Asian Flu" (1957-1958) fluctuated between 1.5 and 4 million. Gatherer (2009) 13 published an estimate of 1.5 million, while Michaelis et al. (2009) published an estimate of two-4 million. Based on a WHO publication, the "Hong Kong Flu" (1968-1969) killed between 1 and 4 million individuals. Michaelis et al. (2009) released a lower estimate of 1-two million. The Russian Flu outbreak of 1977-78 was brought on by precisely the exact same H1N1 virus that caused the Spanish flu. In accordance with Michaelis et al. (2009), around 700,000 died worldwide. What becomes clear from this overview are two things: influenza pandemics are not rare, and the Spanish flu of 1918 was by far the most devastating influenza pandemic in recorded history.

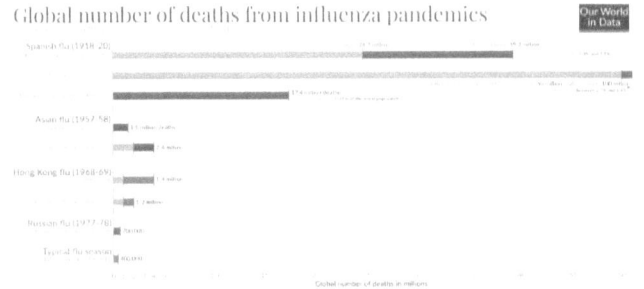

The Effect Of The Spanish Influenza Pandemic On Different Age Groups

This visualization shows the life expectancy in England and Wales by age. The red line indicates the life expectancy for a toddler, together with the lines for revealing how long a person could expect to live once they had reached that given, older, age. The green line, as an instance, signifies the life expectancy. It indicates that life expectancy improved at all ages, meaning the assertion that life expectancy 'just' improved because child mortality diminished isn't correct. This long-term rise of life expectancy at all ages is the focus of this accompanying text here. Related to the flu's effect, it's striking that the research demonstrates that the outbreak had little effect. Even though the life expectancy at ages and at birth dropped by over ten decades, the life expectancy of 60-70-year olds saw no modification. That is at odds with what we'd expect: people that are elderly are most vulnerable to ailments and flu outbreaks. If we take a look at mortality for lower respiratory infections (pneumonia) and upper respiratory ailments now, passing rates are greatest for people who are 70 decades and older. One reason why this pandemic was so devastating was that people accounted for a sizable share of the populace. Were individuals that are elderly resilient to the 1918 pandemic? The research literature indicates that this was true because elderly individuals had lived through a previous flu outbreak -- that the previously discussed 'Russian influenza pandemic' of 1889-90 -- which gave those who lived through it some immunity for the later outbreak of the Spanish flu. The earlier 1889-90 pandemic might have given the older population some immunity, but was a destructive event in itself. According to Smith, 132,000 people died in England, Wales, and Ireland alone.

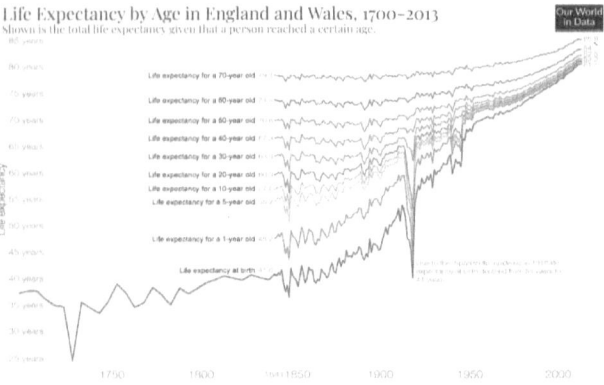

The Lasting Effects Of The 1918 Influenza Pandemic

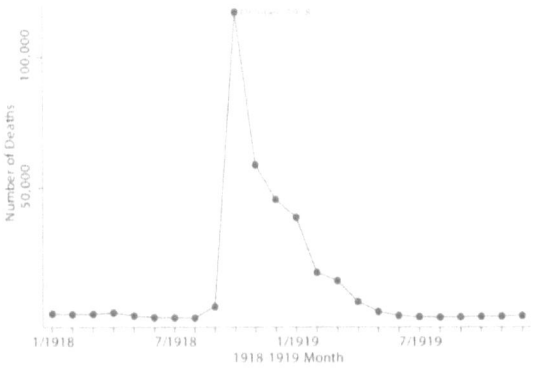

Fig. 1 —U.S. influenza deaths: a, by year; b, by month

I've never put a trigger warning on a post before, but given the current situation, the information here is potentially upsetting to anyone expecting a kid. I don't really feel the present pandemic will probably be as bad as 1918. I am optimistic that the weather will probably operate in our favor, as Tyler contended, America will begin to do the job. Do read my article, What amuses to get a message in 1918-1919? The 1918 flu pandemic struck ferocity in October of 1918 and then over the next four months killed more people than all the US combat deaths of the 20th century. The sudden nature of the pandemic meant that children born just months apart experienced very different conditions in utero. Specifically, children born in 1919 were much more exposed to influenza in utero than children born in 1918 or 1920. The differential to the 1918 flu allows in Is the 1918 Influenza Pandemic Over Douglas Almond test for consequences that are long-term.

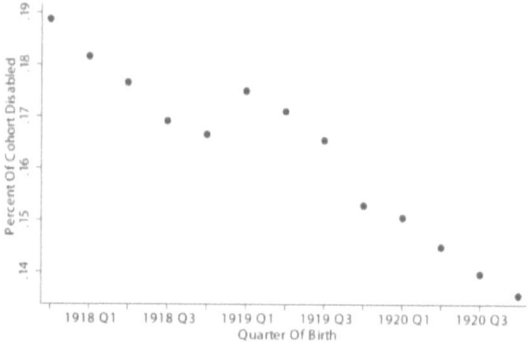

FIG. 2.—1980 male disability rates by quarter of birth: prevented from work by a physical disability.

Almond finds consequences many decades after the exposure. Health is found to affect every outcome. Women and men reveal discontinuous and big discounts in attainment when they'd been through the pandemic in utero. The children of infected mothers were up to 15 percent less likely to graduate from high school. Wages of men were reduced 9 percent due to disease. Socioeconomic status was considerably reduced, and the chance of being poor climbed up to 15 percent contrasted with different cohorts. Entitlement spending has been raised. At appropriate, as an instance, are male handicap rates in 1980, i.e. for men around age 60, by quarter and year of birth. Cohorts born between January and September of 1919 "were in utero in the height of this pandemic and are estimated to get 20 percent greater disability rates at age 61." Figure 3 to right reveals average years of education in 1960; once more the decrease is apparent for people born in 1918. Notice that not all pregnant women contracted flu, so the real effects of flu exposure are bigger, about a 5-month decrease in schooling, largely coming through reduced graduate prices. Education that is reduced and disability translate into government obligations as revealed in the figure below. Almond labels these welfare payments, which might be slightly misleading. These are Social Security Disability payments in 1970. Here Is Almond:

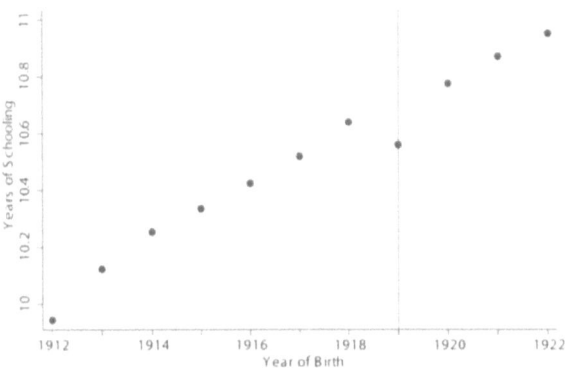

Fig. 3.—1960 average years of schooling: men and women born in the United States

Payments to nonwhites and women in 1970 are plotted in figure 8. The welfare payment was roughly one-third greater for children, or 12 percent greater for girls and nonwhites born in 1919. It's evident that premiums generate these payments to people when we concentrate on the quarter of birth.

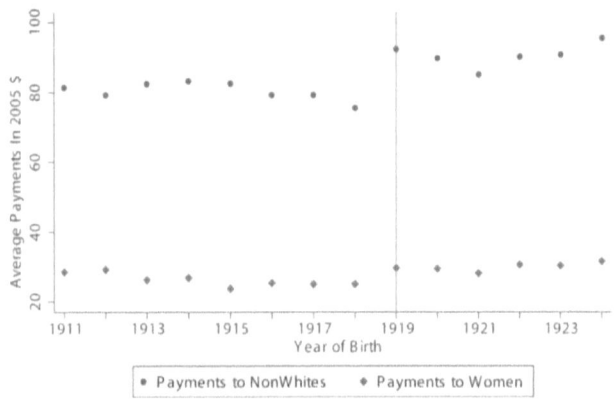

Fig. 8.—Average welfare payments for women and nonwhites: by year of birth

Notice that men and women that were disabled could have dead before 1970, and so these are lower bounds on the disability impact. The 1918 kids, for example, seem about the same as the 1920 kids, so it's not that the flu killed off the weak kids in 1918. Almond was interested in the 1918 pandemic not simply as a historical episode, but to make the case that infant health and infant health programs have a high benefit to cost ratios -- a still relevant lesson.

Chapter - 8 The 1918-19 Vaccine Development And Spanish Influenza Pandemic

When Individuals write about the Spanish Influenza outbreak of 1918-19, they begin with the death toll, the amount of inability of the area, and also individuals that have been infected with the virus. And while those variables were hallmarks of this catastrophic incident, researchers and health workers in the USA and Europe were devising vaccines and immunizing thousands and thousands of individuals in what amounted to medical experimentation on the greatest scale. What exactly were they with? Can they do anything to stop the spread of this illness and to safeguard the immunized? First, in 1918, the US population was 103.2 million. Throughout the 3 waves of the Spanish Influenza outbreak involving spring 1918 and spring 1919, roughly 200 of each 1000 people contracted flu (roughly 20.6 million). Between 0.8 percent (164,800) and 3.1 percent (638,000) of the infected died from flu or pneumonia secondary to it. A couple of vaccines to prevent different diseases were offered at that time-- smallpox vaccine had been utilized for over a hundred years; Louis Pasteur had developed rabies vaccine for post-exposure prophylaxis following an encounter with a rabid animal; typhoid fever vaccines were developed. Diphtheria antitoxin -- a medicine made from infected animals' bloodstream -- was used in the late 1800s for therapy; an early type of diphtheria vaccine was utilized, and cholera vaccines were developed. Almroth Wright had analyzed a vaccine in South African gold miners. Producers marketed and had developed different mixed inventory vaccines of usefulness. At the time, there wasn't a fantastic deal known concerning the understanding of flu as an infectious disease. Medical professionals believed that flu was a communicable disease that was introduced primarily in the winter. Without tools that are specific, cases of flu were hard to differentiate from respiratory disorders. They were able to discover germs, not pathogens.

And scientists and doctors struggled to know whether the annual flu to which they had been used was associated with the prevalent and thoroughly outbreak illness of decades we know was the pandemic flu (1848-49 and 1889-90). German scientist Richard Pfeiffer (1858-1945) claimed to have identified the causative agent of flu in a novel in 1892 -- he also explained rod-shaped bacilli within each event of flu he analyzed. He was able to demonstrate Koch's postulates by inducing the disease in experimental animals. Many specialists accepted his findings and believed Pfeiffer's influenza bacillus because it was accountable for seasonal flu. However, since methods improved, other investigators presented results that conflicted with the findings of Pfeiffer. They discovered his organism in healthy people and people suffering. They looked for Pfeiffer's bacillus in many cases and flu cases, but didn't find it. Though many doctors still thought that Pfeiffer had properly identified the offender, a rising number of others had started to doubt that his findings. Those true believers had any reason to be optimistic that a vaccine might protect against flu as the

108

disease started its next appearance in the USA in early autumn 1918. From October 2, 1918, William H. Park, MD, mind bacteriologist of this New York City Health Department, was operating on a Pfeiffer's germs influenza vaccine. The New York Times reported that Royal S. Copeland, Health Commissioner of New York City, explained the vaccine like a flu preventative and also an "application of an old idea to a new disease." Park was building his vaccine out of heat-killed Pfeiffer's bacilli isolated from sick people and analyzing it on volunteers from Health Department personnel (New York Times, October 2, 1918). Three doses had been given 48 hours. From October 12, he wrote at the New York Medical Journal that he had been vaccinating workers from big businesses and soldiers in military camps. He expected to have proof to demonstrate the efficacy of the vaccine in a couple of months (Park WH, 1918).

In November, the Newark Evening News reported that 39,000 Doses of Leary-Park flu vaccine was prepared and doses had been used. (Timothy Leary was a professor at Tufts University School of Medicine.) Even though it was too soon to tell whether the vaccine was successful,". . . the average individual need not have any fear of the vaccine's outcomes. Neurotic and rheumatic people, nevertheless, seem to be more sensitive to the vaccine, while kids accept it with less interference than adults" (Newark Evening News, 1918). From December 13, 1918, Copeland wasn't so convinced about his section vaccine. He told the Times that vaccines produced from the bacilli of Pfeiffer seemed to have no impact on flu prevention. Instead, he was convinced that a combined bacterial vaccine (streptococcal, pneumococcal, staphylococcal, and Pfeiffer's bacilli) developed by E.C. Rosenow in the Mayo Foundation was a powerful preventative. And while he believed that many individuals in New York had been subjected to Spanish flu, he said he could have Park prepare a number of their Rosenow vaccines to immunize individuals in New York through winter (New York Times, December 13, 1918). Well over 500,000 doses of Rosenow vaccine were created (Eyler, 2009).Tulane University, University of Pittsburgh, as well as personal doctors, were creating their vaccines. Convalescent serum was also utilized (Boston Post, January 6, 1919; Robertson & Koehler, 1918). The Deseret (UT) Evening News mentioned on December 14, 1918, that free vaccine was first available in communities across the nation. According to my survey of paper and recent clinical journal articles, it's apparent that lots of hundreds of thousands, maybe even a thousand or even more, doses of vaccines have been generated during the pandemic decades. (A couple of years back I wrote another blog article about Rosenow's vaccine) The Editorial Committee of the American Journal of Public Health attempted to place a damper on people's expectations concerning the vaccines. They composed in January 1919 the causative organism of this present influenza was unknown, and so the vaccines being generated had just an opportunity in being targeted at the ideal target. They noticed that vaccines for secondary ailments made a sense, but all the vaccines being generated have to be seen as experimental. Acknowledging the somewhat ad hoc character vaccine development from the present crisis, they advocated that management classes be utilized with the vaccines, which the differences between experimental and control group be lessened, as to the threat of exposure, time of exposure during the outbreak, etc (Editorial Committee of the American Journal of Public Health, 1919).

Surely none of the vaccines' viral flu infection -- we understand today that flu is brought on by a virus, and not one of the vaccines protected against it. But were any of these protective from the bacterial diseases that developed secondary to flu? Vaccinologist Stanley A. Plotkin, MD, believes that they weren't. He advised us: "The bacterial vaccines designed for Spanish flu were probably ineffective since at the time it wasn't understood that pneumococcal bacteria come in many, several serotypes and of their bacterial group they predicted B. influenza, just 1 form is a significant pathogen." To put it differently, the vaccine programmers had little capability to identify, isolate, and create all of the possible disease-causing strains of germs circulating at the moment. Now there's a pneumococcal vaccine for kids that protects against 13 serotypes of the germs, along with the vaccine for adults shields against 23 serotypes. A 2010 informative article, however, describes a meta-analysis of bacterial vaccine research from 1918-19 and indicates a more positive interpretation. According to the 13 studies that met inclusion criteria, the authors conclude that a few of the vaccines might have decreased the assault speed of pneumonia following viral flu infection. They imply that regardless of the restricted quantities of bacteria strains from the vaccines, vaccination might have resulted in cross-protection from multiple associated breeds (Chien, 2010). It wasn't until the 1930s that investigators

111

established that the flu was brought on by a virus, not a bacterium. Pfeiffer's flu bacillus would finally be termed Haemophilus influenzae, the title keeping the heritage of its longstanding, though incorrect, association with flu. And now, flu vaccines -- also as H. influenzae type b vaccines – are broadly available to reduce disease.

Influenza Vaccine

Influenza vaccines, also known as flu shots or influenza jabs, are compounds that protect against infection by influenza viruses. New variations of these vaccines have been developed twice annually since the flu virus immediately changes. Even though their effectiveness varies from year to year, many supply modest to high security against flu. The United States Centers for Disease Control and Prevention (CDC) estimates that vaccination against flu reduces illness, clinical visits, hospitalizations, and deaths. Immunized employees, who do catch the flu, come back to work half a day earlier on average. Vaccine efficacy in people under two years old and people over 65 years old remains unclear because of a shortage of high excellent research. Vaccinating kids can protect those around them.

The World Health Organization (WHO) and the U.S. Centers for Disease Control and Prevention (CDC) recommend yearly vaccination for almost all people over age six months, particularly those at high risk. The European Centre for Disease Prevention and Control (ECDC) additionally urges annual vaccination for these high-risk groups: pregnant women, the elderly, and children between six months and five decades old, those with specific health issues, and people who are employed in health care.

The vaccines are safe. Fever occurs in five to ten percent of children vaccinated. Muscle aches or feelings of fatigue may occur. At a speed of approximately one case per million doses, the vaccine was associated with a rise in

Guillain syndrome among individuals in certain years. They are suggested that flu vaccines are generated using eggs. Influenza vaccines aren't recommended in those who've experienced a serious allergy to versions of the vaccine. The vaccine comes from diminished forms that are viral and dormant. The weakened vaccine in individuals with a weakened immune system, children, adults, or recommended in pregnant women. Based upon the kind they are sometimes injected into a muscle, then sprayed into the nose, or inserted into the center of skin (intradermal). The vaccine wasn't available throughout 2018-2019 and 2019-2020 flu seasons. Vaccination against the flu started in the 1930s. It's about the List of Essential Medicines, the most powerful and best medicines of the World Health Organization. The wholesale cost in the developing world is roughly US $5.25 per dose as of 2014. In the USA, the vaccine prices less than US$25 as part of 2015, each dose.

Medical Uses

The U.S Centers for Disease Control and Prevention (CDC) urges the flu vaccine in order to stop its spread and protect individuals. When someone buys, anxiety that the vaccine didn't contain the influenza vaccine may decrease the severity of influenza. It requires about two weeks after vaccination for antibodies that are protective to form. A 2012 meta-analysis discovered that influenza vaccination was successful 67 percent of their time; the inhabitants that benefited the most were HIV-positive adults aged 18 to 55 (76 percent), healthy adults aged 18 to 46 (roughly 70 percent), and wholesome children aged six to 24 months (66 percent). The flu vaccine also seems to protect against myocardial infarction using a benefit of 15 to 45 percent.

Effectiveness

There is a vaccine evaluated by its effectiveness -- the extent to which It reduces its efficacy -- the reduction in risk after the vaccine is put into use -- and also a risk of disorder under controlled conditions. In the event of flu, since it's quantified utilizing the degrees efficacy it is forecasted to be lower. Influenza vaccines show efficacy. Yet, studies on the efficacy of influenza vaccines in the actual world are hard; vaccines could be imperfectly coordinated, virus incidence varies widely between years, and flu can be confused with other influenza-like ailments. But in most years (16 of those 19 years earlier 2007), the influenza vaccine strains are a fantastic match for its circulating strains, and even a mismatched vaccine could frequently offer cross-protection. The virus varies due to drift, a mutation in the virus which is responsible for a breed. Yearly influenza vaccination that is repeated offers you constant protection against flu. There's indicative evidence that repeated vaccinations might make a decrease in vaccine efficacy for specific flu subtypes; this does not have any significance to present recommendations for annual vaccinations but may influence future vaccination coverage. As of 2019, a vaccine is recommended by the CDC since studies reveal the efficacy of influenza vaccination.

Criticism

Influenza vaccines have predicted clinical signs concerning influenza vaccines "rap" and has consequently declared them to be unsuccessful; it's known for esophageal clinical trials, which many in the area maintain as unethical. Institutions such as the CDC and the National Institutes of Health, also from key figures in the area such as Anthony Fauci reject his perspectives on the effectiveness of influenza vaccines. Michael Osterholm, who headed the Center for Infectious Disease Research and Policy 2012 review on influenza vaccines, advocated getting the vaccine but criticized its promotion, stating, "We've over-promoted and overhyped this particular vaccine... it doesn't shield as encouraged. It is a sales job: it is all public relations."

Kids

The CDC recommends that everybody except babies under the age of six months must get the seasonal flu vaccine. Vaccination campaigns generally focus particular attention on individuals that are at elevated risk of severe complications if they catch the flu, such as elderly women, kids under 59 weeks, the elderly, and individuals with chronic illnesses or weakened immune systems, in addition to individuals to whom they are vulnerable, such as healthcare workers. Since the departure rate is too high among babies who catch flu, the CDC and the WHO recommend that household contacts and caregivers of babies be vaccinated to decrease the danger of passing a flu infection to the baby. In children, the vaccine seems to lower the chance of potential disease and flu. In children under the age of 2, information is constrained. Throughout 2017-18 flu season, the CDC manager suggested that 85 percent of those kids who died "probably weren't vaccinated." In the USA, in January 2019, the CDC recommends that children aged six through 35 months can receive either 0.25 milliliters or 0.5 milliliters per dose of Fluzone Quadrivalent. There's not any preference for one of the dose quantity of Fluzone Quadrivalent for this age category. All men 36 weeks of age and older must get 0.5 milliliters per dose of Fluzone Quadrivalent. In October 2018, Afluria Quadrivalent is accredited for children six months old and older from the United States Children six months through 35 months old should get 0.25 milliliters for every dose of Afluria Quadrivalent. All men 36 weeks of age and older must get 0.5 milliliters per dose of Afluria Quadrivalent. As of February 2018, Afluria Tetra is accredited for children and adults five decades old and older in Canada. In 2014, the Canadian National Advisory Committee on Immunization (NACI) released an overview of flu vaccination in healthy 5-18-year-olds, also in 2015, printed a report on using pediatric Fluad in kids 6-72 weeks old.

16 percent get symptoms like the flu, adults, while about 10 percent of adults do. Vaccination decreased confirmed cases of flu from roughly 2.4 percent to 1.1 percent. No impact on the operation was discovered. In adults, a review from the Cochrane Collaboration found without impacting transmission or influenza-related complications that hepatitis led to days lost and a reduction in both flu symptoms. In healthy functioning adults, flu vaccines may offer mild protection from virologically- confirmed influenza, although such defense is significantly diminished or absent in certain seasons. In healthcare employees, a benefit was discovered by a 2006 evaluation. Of the studies in this review, just two also evaluated the relationship of individual mortality relative to employees flu vaccine uptake; equally discovered that greater rates of healthcare employee vaccination associated with decreased patient deaths. A 2014 review found advantages to patients when healthcare employees were immunized, as encouraged by moderate signs predicated in part on the observed reduction in all-cause deaths in patients that their healthcare employees were granted immunization compared in comparison to patients in which the employees weren't provided disease.

Mature

Evidence for an effect in adults more than 65 years old is unclear. Systematic reviews analyzing the case and controlled, control studies found that a deficiency of signs that is high quality. Reviews of the case-control studies found effects against flu, pneumonia, and death. The older, the group most vulnerable to flu, benefits from the embryo. There are reasons for this decrease in vaccine efficiency, the most frequent of which would be associated with age and the immunological role. In a non-pandemic calendar year, an individual in the USA aged 50-64 is almost ten times more likely to die an influenza-associated departure than a younger man, and a man over age 65 is more than ten times more likely to die an influenza-associated departure compared to 50-64 age category. An influenza vaccine is formulated to offer a more powerful immune reaction. Evidence suggests that vaccinating the elderly leads to the vaccine. An influenza vaccine comprising an adjuvant was accepted by the U.S. Food and Drug Administration (FDA) in November 2015, to be used by adults aged 65 decades old and older. The vaccine is promoted as Fluad from the U.S. and was available in the 2016-2017 flu period. The vaccine includes the MF59C.1 adjuvant that is an oil-in-water emulsion of squalene oil. It's the seasonal influenza vaccine. It isn't clear if there's a substantial advantage for the elderly to utilize an influenza vaccine comprising the MF59C.1 adjuvant. Fluad may be utilized as an alternate approved for individuals 65 decades and older. It is advocated to decrease flu outbreaks in these people. Even though there's absolutely no evidence from trials that healthcare employees help protect older people, there is evidence of advantage.

Chapter - 9 Lessons In The 1918 Spanish Flu Pandemic

MONDAY, April 20, 2020 (Health Day News) -- "The virus struck dread since it murdered tens of thousands and sickened millions -- and today the 1918 influenza pandemic provides courses. "The questions they asked then are the questions being asked today," explained Christopher Nichols, an associate professor of history at Oregon State University, in Corvallis. "And while it is very rare that background gives a simple straightforward lesson to the current, this is one of these cases." Experts say that there are four important takeaways in 1918.

Here is the first:

"As devastating as the present pandemic could be, the Spanish influenza pandemic is still the worst in history," said E. Thomas Ewing, a history professor at Virginia Tech in Blacksburg. From now three waves of influenza swept across the world at least 50 million people have been dead. In contrast, influenza pandemics in 1957, 1968, and 2009 maintained an estimated total of 225,000 Americans and 3 million individuals worldwide.)

Here is the 2nd:

There are differences between the COVID-19 and 1918 pandemic. "Afterward they did not even know that it was a virus," Ewing said. "There'd been years of research about microbes, so that they knew that it had been moved person-to-person through respiratory drops, by coughing and sneezing. But viruses were not found until the 1930s since they did not have strong enough microscopes." Because of this, testing was difficult to find. It did not exist. Influenza-caused disorders were more infectious than COVID-19 and were much more deadly, Nichols explained. And that presents the best threat to older influenza. "It influenced everyone old and young," Nichols explained. "However, it killed the safest one of people: an all-American 22-year-old soccer player. Individuals in their prime got struck down. So, the panic that animated men and women in the autumn of 1918 were different."

Here is the 3rd:

Despite these differences, 2020 is striking. There was no cure for the disease and no vaccine a healthcare system might decode. And here is takeaway No. 4: In both pandemics, the best immediate response was -- and is social distancing, Nichols explained. "It was known as crowding' control back then," he explained. "However, whatever you call it, restricting contact functioned in 1918 -- and it functions now." Along with distancing and the comprehensive closures are set into position, the faster a pandemic could be brought under control, Nichols added. People who lived through influenza discovered that lesson the hard way, based on Carolyn Orban in Columbia.

"Like pandemics, in 1918 you had stress between biological truth and socioeconomic fact," she explained. "Biology isn't changeable. But behavior is. Yes, social distancing was a thing in 1918, also in which it had been practiced, it worked."

However mistrust, from fear, fear interests -- and even boredom many were fast to jump ship and slow to have on board. Historians see the signs in letters written in precisely the time by the families. "The mom is saying, 'We all must be patient, lay low and wait it out,' while the kid is saying she has had enough of no faculty and no friends, and she is planning a Halloween celebration, in the same way, the maximum amount of deaths are occurring," Orban clarified. That tension helps clarify the lack of a strong and ancient reaction according to Ewing and Nichols. Officials stalled for a while and played down the danger. Why? Some motives were exceptional to 1918.

"The hay strike throughout a critical phase of World War I," Nichols explained. "From the time the initial presumed U.S. instance was identified in March 1918 in a Kansas army foundation, there was great concern about soldiers becoming ill. That issue was well-founded: Army camps' quarters were dishes for sickness," Orban explained.

"Boys will... return in body bags in these amounts that finally it became nearly impossible to distinguish the war effort from the pandemic," she explained. And early on, the authorities had the reason Nichols mentioned. Flu deaths were reduced and tens of thousands of troops were led into the front lines in Europe. "The focus is completely on the last major push to finish the war," he clarified. So, the information from Washington, D.C., back then may seem familiar now: Do not panic. It is no big thing. "Initially they inform the public it is not a large issue, or even -- as its name implies -- that it is a foreign disorder that only affects 'other people.'

Conclusion

Nichols said, "It was not until the autumn, following a more virulent type of Spanish influenza had emerged, that Washington, D.C., obtained rough. Meanwhile, the lack of a federal reaction left states and cities to go off by themselves and make decisions for them." Nichols said the market was chosen by many plus distancing is placing off by them, together with outcomes. Many others didn't while cities such as Seattle and San Francisco ordered people to wear masks when they had been out in public. Colleges never shut, asserting that they were cleaner. Many cities failed, although October 1918, when deaths started to skyrocket. According to Ewing, "There were lots of inconsistencies." Two studies published at the Proceedings of the National Academy of Sciences in 2007 looked at the impact of health measures, such as business-hour limitations, mask legislation, along with the shuttering of dancing halls and colleges, theaters, and churches in over 15 cities in 1918. Both studies found that towns which acted most forcefully -- such as St. Louis, that imposed a near-complete lockdown in two weeks of its initial Spanish influenza instance -- had considerably lower summit departure rates than towns which hedged their bets -- such as New Orleans, Boston, and Philadelphia. The point isn't so social networking is a complete panacea, but there's no "business-as-usual throughout a pandemic," Nichols explained.

So the lesson of 1918 is apparent: "If people's wellness is the principal focus, then eliminate that from your head,"

Nichols said. "Spanish influenza informs us that social networking works. It works best when we act and adhere together -- and base our conclusions not on social or financial issues, but data, science, and details.